ULTIMATE
SPORTS
NUTRITION

Ellen Coleman, RD, MA, MPH

Nutrition Consultant,
The Sport Clinic,
Riverside, California

Suzanne Nelson Steen, DSc, RD

University of Washington,
Department of Intercollegiate Athletics,
Husky Sports Nutrition Services

Bull Publishing Company
Palo Alto, California

Copyright © 2000 Bull Publishing Company

Bull Publishing Company
P.O. Box 208
Palo Alto, CA 94302-0208
Phone: (650) 322-2855 / FAX: (650) 327-3300
www.bullpub.com

ISBN: 0-923521-56-9

Distributed to the trade by:
Publishers Group West
1700 Fourth Street
Berkeley, CA 94710

Library of Congress Cataloging-in-Publication Data
Coleman, Ellen
    Ultimate sports nutrition / by Ellen Coleman, Suzanne Nelson Steen.
2nd ed.
        p. cm.
    Rev. ed. of: The ultimate sports nutrition handbook. c1996.
    Includes bibliographical references and index.
    ISBN 0-923521-56-9
    1. Athletes—Nutrition—Handbooks, manuals, etc. I. Steen, Suzanne
Nelson. II. Coleman, Ellen. Ultimate sports nutrition handbook. III.
Title.

TX361.A8 C56 2000
613.2'024'796—dc21   00-056486

Manufactured in the United States of America

Publisher: James Bull
Cover Design: Robb Pawlak, Pawlak Design
Interior Design and Composition:
Dianne Nelson, Shadow Canyon Graphics

Third printing

*Dedicated to
David Bull—
an athlete, scholar,
and friend*

CONTENTS

LIST OF TABLES

LIST OF FIGURES

1

NUTRIENTS: BUILDING BLOCKS FOR PERFORMANCE

Three primary factors influence your athletic performance: genetics, training, and nutrition. You can't do anything about your heredity, but you do have control over your training and food choices.

Many athletes who train hard to excel are defeated by their diets instead of their competitors. Although a balanced diet won't guarantee you athletic success, an unbalanced diet may undermine your training.

Some athletes will try any dietary regimen in an effort to improve performance, stay healthy, or lose weight. The desire for that elusive "secret ingredient" can cause them to disregard sound nutrition practices and become victims of nutrition fraud. Most popular diets and supplements don't give athletes the results they want, and some dietary fads are harmful.

Choosing the proper food is as important to your athletic success as having the most appropriate training program. There are sound dietary strategies that you can use to perform closer to your potential. **Ultimate Sports Nutrition** provides the most current information on nutrition for peak athletic performance. It presents sensible nutrition advice that you can put into practice immediately.

NUTRIENTS

Food fulfills three basic needs:

1. It provides energy.
2. It supports new tissue growth and tissue repair.
3. It helps to regulate metabolism.

These three requirements are met by components of foods called **nutrients**. There are six classes of nutrients, and each class has special chemical characteristics suited to meet the specific needs of the body. The six classes are carbohydrates, fats, proteins, vitamins, minerals, and water.

Carbohydrates

Carbohydrates, such as sugar and starch, are the most readily available source of food energy. During digestion and metabolism, all carbohydrates are eventually broken down to the simple sugar **glucose** for use as the body's principal energy source. Glucose is stored in the muscles and liver as a substance called **glycogen**, which is a long chain of glucose molecules hooked together. A high-carbohydrate diet is necessary to maintain muscle glycogen—the primary fuel for most sports. The importance of carbohydrate for peak performance is discussed in Chapters 2 and 5.

Sugar and starch are grouped together as carbohydrates because they have a chemical similarity. All carbohydrates are made up of one or more simple sugars, the three most common being glucose, fructose, and galactose. The simple sugar glucose connected to fructose forms sucrose, or table sugar. When more than two glucose molecules are connected, they become a starch, or complex carbohydrate. Starches contain anywhere from 300 to 1,000 or more glucose units hooked together.

Although our bodies use both the sugars and starches for energy, a high-performance diet emphasizes **nutrient-dense** carbohydrates. Nutrient-dense carbohydrates such as whole-grain breads and cereals, rice, beans, pasta, vegetables, and fruits supply other nutrients such as vitamins, minerals, protein, and fiber. Sweet foods that are high in sugar (candy bars, donuts, and cookies) supply carbohydrate, but they also contain a high amount of fat and only insignificant amounts of vitamins and minerals.

Fruit contains the sweetest of all simple sugars—fructose. Since fruit is mostly water, its sugar and calorie content is relatively low. Like starchy foods, most fruits are rich in nutrients and virtually fat-free.

Fats

Fats, or lipids, are the most concentrated source of food energy. One gram of fat supplies about nine calories, compared to the four calories per gram supplied by carbohydrate and protein. Fats are the body's only source of the **essential fatty acids** linoleic and linolenic acid that are required for growth, healthy skin, and healthy hair. Fat insulates and protects the body's organs against trauma and exposure to cold. Fats are also involved in the absorption and transport of the fat-soluble vitamins.

Fatty acids are divided into two categories—**saturated** and **unsaturated** (including polyunsaturated and monounsaturated fatty acids). These fatty acids differ from each other chemically based on the nature of the bond between carbon and hydrogen atoms.

As a general rule, saturated fat (butter and lard) is solid at room temperature and is derived mainly from animal sources. Unsaturated fat (e.g., safflower, canola, and corn oil) is liquid at room temperature and found mainly in plant sources. Palm and coconut oils are exceptions—they are highly saturated vegetable fats. Saturated fat should be restricted because it raises blood cholesterol, which in turn increases the risk of heart disease. The relationship between dietary fat and heart disease is discussed in Chapters 2 and 7.

Proteins

Protein is a major structural component of all body tissues and is required for tissue growth and repair. Proteins are necessary components of hormones, enzymes, and blood plasma transport systems. Protein is not a significant energy source during rest or exercise. However, the body will use protein for energy if you're not eating enough calories or carbohydrates (during starvation or a low-carbohydrate diet).

The proteins in both animal and plant foods are composed of structural units called **amino acids**. Of the more than twenty amino acids that have been identified, nine must be provided by our diet and are called **essential amino acids,** as shown in Table 1-1. Meat, fish, dairy products, eggs, and poultry contain all nine essential amino acids and are called **complete proteins.** Vegetable proteins, such as beans and grains, are called **incomplete proteins** because they do not supply all the essential amino acids.

The body can make complete proteins if a variety of plant foods—beans, grains, vegetables, fruits, nuts, and seeds—and sufficient calories are eaten during the day. Since the body utilizes amino acids from foods eaten at different meals, vegetarians don't need to combine specific foods within a meal to obtain complete proteins. Well-balanced vegetarian diets may even decrease the risk of heart disease and cancer, because they are lower in fat and higher in nutrient-dense carbohydrates than the average American diet.

TABLE 1-1
Proteins (Essential Amino Acids)

Isoleucine	Methionine	Tryptophan
Leucine	Phenylalanine	Valine
Lysine	Threonine	Histidine

Vitamins

Vitamins are organic molecules (they contain carbon) that the body cannot manufacture but which it requires in small amounts. Contrary to what many people believe, vitamins do not provide energy. They are metabolic regulators that help govern the processes of energy production, growth, maintenance, and repair. Thirteen vitamins have been identified; each has a specific function in the body and also works in complicated ways with other nutrients. The function and sources of most of the vitamins are shown in Table 1-2.

Vitamins are divided into two groups: **water soluble** and **fat soluble**. Fat-soluble vitamins include A, D, E, and K. They are stored in body fat, principally in the liver. Taking a greater amount of vitamins A and D than the body needs over a period of time can produce serious toxic effects. Too much vitamin A can cause loss of appetite, headaches, irritability, liver damage, bone pain, and neurological problems, including brain damage. Too much vitamin D can cause weight loss, vomiting, irritability, destructive deposits of excess calcium in soft tissues (like the kidneys and lungs), and potentially fatal kidney failure.

While vitamin A is found only in animals, dark orange-yellow and green leafy plants contain substances called carotenes (e.g., beta-carotene) that your body can convert to vitamin A. Unlike vitamin A, carotene is fairly safe when consumed in large amounts. The body stores excesses of carotenes (which can make the skin look yellow-orange) rather than converting them to vitamin A.

Vitamin C and the B complex vitamins are soluble in water and must be replaced on a regular basis. When you consume more water-soluble vitamins than you need, the excess is eliminated in the urine. Although this increases the vitamin content of your urine, it doesn't help your performance. Consuming excessive amounts of water-soluble vitamins, such as niacin and B_6, can also cause dangerous side effects (see Chapter 8).

TABLE 1-2
U.S. Dietary Reference Intakes for Vitamins

NUTRIENT	FUNCTIONS	SOURCES
Vitamin C	Collagen formation, immunity, antioxidant	Citrus fruits, tomatoes, strawberries, potatoes, broccoli, cabbage
Vitamin B_1 (Thiamin)	Energy production, central nervous system	Meat, whole-grain cereals, milk, beans
Niacin	Energy production, synthesis of fat and amino acids	Peanut butter, whole-grain cereals, greens, meat, poultry, fish
Vitamin B_6	Protein metabolism, hemoglobin synthesis, energy production	Whole-grain cereals, bananas, meat, spinach, cabbage, lima beans
Folacin	New cell growth, red blood cell production	Greens, mushrooms, liver
Vitamin B_{12} (Cobalamin)	Energy metabolism, red blood cell production, central nervous system	Animal foods
Vitamin A	Vision, skin, antioxidant, immunity	Milk, egg yolk, liver, yogurt, carrots, greens
Vitamin D	Formation of bones, aids absorption of calcium	Sunlight, fortified dairy products, eggs, fish
Vitamin E	Antioxidant, protects unsaturated fats in cells from damage	Vegetable oils, margarines, grains
Vitamin K	Blood clotting	Greens, liver

To find the DRI for a specific nutrient, search the National Academies of Sciences web page. The URL is: http://www.4.nationalacademies.org/news.nsf

Minerals

Minerals are inorganic compounds (they don't contain carbon) that serve a variety of functions in the body. Some minerals, such as calcium and phosphorus, are used to build bones and teeth. Others are important components of hormones, such as iodine in thyroxin. Iron is crucial in the formation of hemoglobin, the oxygen carrier within red blood cells. The function and sources of most of the minerals are shown in Table 1-3.

Minerals also contribute to a number of the body's regulatory functions. These include regulation of muscle contraction, conduction of nerve impulses, clotting of blood, and regulation of normal heart rhythm.

Minerals are classified into two groups based on the body's need. **Major minerals,** such as calcium, are needed in amounts greater than 100 milligrams per day. **Minor minerals,** or trace elements, such as iron, are required in amounts less than 100 milligrams per day. Calcium and iron are both important minerals for athletes, especially women, and are discussed in Chapter 8.

Water

Water is the most essential of all nutrients for athletes. An adequate supply of water is necessary for control of body temperature (especially during exercise), for energy production, and for elimination of waste products from metabolism.

Dehydration—the loss of body water—impairs athletic performance and increases the risk of heat illnesses (heat exhaustion and heatstroke). Water is probably the nutrient most neglected by athletes.

It's easy to overlook the benefits of water because it is so readily available and inexpensive. The importance of proper fluid replacement for optimal performance is discussed in Chapter 9.

TABLE 1-3
U.S. Dietary Reference Intakes for Minerals

NUTRIENT	FUNCTIONS	SOURCES
Calcium	Bone formation, enzyme reactions, muscle contractions	Dairy products, green leafy vegetables, beans
Iron	Hemoglobin formation, muscle growth and function, energy production	Lean meat, beans, dried fruit, some green leafy vegetables
Magnesium	Energy production, muscle relaxation, nerve conduction	Grains, nuts, meats, beans
Sodium	Nerve impulses, muscle action, body fluid balance	Table salt, small amounts in most food except fruit
Potassium	Fluid balance, muscle action, glycogen and protein synthesis	Bananas, orange juice, fruits, vegetables
Zinc	Tissue growth and healing, immunity, gonadal development	Meat, shellfish, oysters, grains
Copper	Hemoglobin formation, energy production, immunity	Whole grains, beans, nuts dried fruit, shellfish
Selenium	Antioxidant, protects against free radicals, enhances vitamin E	Meat, seafood, grains
Chromium	Part of glucose tolerance factor—helps insulin	Whole grains, meat, cheese, beer
Manganese	Bone and tissue development, fat synthesis	Nuts, grains, beans, tea, fruits, vegetables
Iodine	Regulates metabolism	Iodized salt, seafood
Fluoride	Formation of bones and tooth enamel	Tap water, tea, coffee, rice, spinach, lettuce
Phosphorus	Builds bones and teeth, metabolism	Meat, fish, dairy products, carbonated drinks

To find the DRI for a specific nutrient, search the National Academies of Sciences web page. The URL is: http://www.4.nationalacademies.org/news.nsf

Variety, Moderation, and Balance

There are three basic principles to follow when choosing foods to obtain a high-performance diet:

- **Variety** refers to eating foods from each of the five food groups daily, as well as different foods within each group. No one food or supplement provides all the nutrients required for health and performance.
- **Moderation** means not eating too little or too much of any one food or nutrient.
- **Balance,** which results from moderation and variety, requires an appropriate intake of essential nutrients. It also refers to balancing calorie intake and energy expenditure to maintain a healthy weight or body composition.

For peak performance, athletes need to eat a varied diet most of the time. You can't just focus on your pre-exercise meal or what you eat the day before competition.

While variety is important, don't be overly concerned if you occasionally deviate from a balanced diet. Obtaining a balanced diet isn't as hard as the supplement salespeople would have you believe.

NUTRIENTS AND PEAK PERFORMANCE

Of the 40 known nutrients, 10 are considered **leader nutrients.** If you obtain adequate amounts of leader nutrients from the foods you eat, you probably will obtain the other 30 nutrients as well.

The 10 leader nutrients are protein, carbohydrate, fat, vitamin A, vitamin C, thiamin, riboflavin, niacin, calcium, and iron. The five food groups in the Food Guide Pyramid (discussed in the next chapter) were developed based on these leader nutrients. The foods in the grain group are high in carbohydrate, thiamin, niacin, and iron. The fruit and vegetable groups contain foods high in vitamins A and C. Meat group foods are high in protein, niacin, iron, and thiamin. Foods in the milk group are good sources of calcium, riboflavin, and protein.

Since no one food or food group supplies all the nutrients you need, it's important to choose a wide variety of foods from the five groups in the Pyramid. By eating at least the minimum number of servings from each food group daily, you can be reasonably assured you're getting the nutrients you need for optimal performance. The next chapter discusses how to develop a training meal plan to get the most out of your workouts.

2

TRAINING DIETS FOR PERFORMANCE AND HEALTH

E ventually almost all athletes will encounter problems due to haphazard or irregular eating habits. Nutrition-related diffi- culties are usually due to inadequate carbohydrate intake and may result in reduced speed, impaired endurance, and diffi- culty concentrating. Unwanted weight loss or weight gain may also be the result of poor food choices. Sound eating habits can help to prevent these problems and promote optimal perform- ance. A healthy diet should also help to prevent major health problems—heart disease, certain cancers, diabetes, stroke, and osteoporosis.

There is no single diet for athletes, since each sport makes nutritional demands that require individual attention for peak performance (see Chapter 4). However, the nutritional guidelines developed to promote health establish a good foundation for athletes who desire peak performance. This chapter discusses these guidelines and how they make up a training diet for ath- letes and active people. The nutritional requirements for specific sports are addressed in later chapters.

FOOD GUIDE PYRAMID

The **Food Guide Pyramid** (Figure 2-1) shows the foods that should be included in a healthful diet and in what amounts. The grain group forms the base of the pyramid, the fruit and vegetable groups are on the second tier, and the meat and dairy groups are on the third tier. Since fats and sweets should be consumed in limited amounts, these items are grouped in a small section at the top of the pyramid. Alcoholic beverages are also part of this group. Fats, sweets, and alcohol are often called "empty calories" because they are high in calories but low in most nutrients.

FIGURE 2-1.
The Food Guide Pyramid

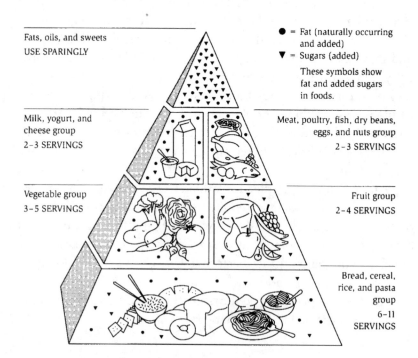

Fats, oils, and sweets
USE SPARINGLY

● = Fat (naturally occurring and added)
▼ = Sugars (added)

These symbols show fat and added sugars in foods.

Milk, yogurt, and cheese group
2–3 SERVINGS

Meat, poultry, fish, dry beans, eggs, and nuts group
2–3 SERVINGS

Vegetable group
3–5 SERVINGS

Fruit group
2–4 SERVINGS

Bread, cereal, rice, and pasta group
6–11 SERVINGS

Americans, and particularly athletes, should be eating heartily from the grain, vegetable, and fruit groups since these groups have the highest recommended number of servings and are nutrient-rich sources of carbohydrate. Table 2-1 indicates what counts as one serving from each group.

TABLE 2-1
What Counts as One Serving?

BREAD, CEREAL, RICE, AND PASTA GROUP
1 slice bread
½ cup cooked rice or pasta
½ cup cooked cereal
1 oz ready-to-eat cereal

VEGETABLE GROUP
½ cup chopped raw or cooked vegetables
1 cup leafy raw vegetables
1/2 cup tomato or vegetable juice

FRUIT GROUP
1 piece fruit or melon wedge
¾ cup juice
½ cup canned fruit
¼ cup dried fruit

MILK, YOGURT, AND CHEESE GROUP
1 cup milk or yogurt
1½ oz natural cheese
2 oz processed cheese

MEAT, POULTRY, FISH, DRY BEANS, EGGS, AND NUTS GROUP
2½–3 oz cooked lean meat, poultry, or fish
½ cup cooked beans, or 1 egg, or 2 tbsp. peanut butter as 1 oz lean meat

FATS, OILS, AND SWEETS
Use sparingly, *especially if you need to lose weight.*

The amount you eat may be more than one serving. For example, a dinner portion of spaghetti would count as 2 or 3 servings.

TABLE 2-2
How Many Servings Do You Need Each Day?

Calorie Level*	Women and Some Older Adults	Children, Teen Girls, Active Women, Most Men	Teen Boys and Active Men
	About 1,600	About 2,200	About 2,800
Bread Group	6	9	11
Vegetable Group	3	4	5
Fruit Group	2	3	4
Milk Group	2–3**	2–3**	2–3**
Meat Group	2	2	3
	for a total of 5 ounces	for a total of 6 ounces	for a total of 7 ounces

* These are the calorie levels if you choose low-fat, leanfoods from the 5 major food groups and use foods from the fats, oils, and sweets group sparingly.
** Women who are pregnant or breast-feeding, teenagers, and young adults to age 24 need 3 servings.

Source: U.S. Department of Agriculture and the U.S. Department of Health and Human Services.

The number of calories the Food Guide Pyramid provides will vary, depending on the selection of foods within the groups and the number of servings eaten (see Table 2-2). The minimum number of servings from the Food Guide Pyramid provides about 1,600 calories if you choose low-fat, lean foods from the five groups and use items from the fats and sweets group sparingly. Eating the minimum number of servings from the Pyramid will promote body fat loss for most athletes while providing adequate nutrients. High-calorie items such as fats, sweets, and alcohol should be limited when body fat reduction is desired. Effective strategies for body fat loss are discussed in Chapter 11.

Consuming the maximum number of servings (with a limited intake of fats and sweets) provides about 2,800 calories. Athletes who have higher calorie needs for weight maintenance or weight gain can eat a greater number of servings from the food groups by eating between-meal snacks. Emphasis should be placed on the grain, fruit, and vegetable groups since they generally provide more carbohydrate and less fat than the meat and milk groups. There's also no harm in eating a reasonable amount of sweets to supply needed calories once nutrient needs have been met. Effective strategies for weight gain are discussed in Chapter 11.

DIETARY GUIDELINES FOR AMERICANS

The Dietary Guidelines are designed to help Americans choose diets that will promote health, reduce chronic disease risks, support active lives, and meet nutrient requirements. The Food Guide Pyramid is based on these recommendations. The guidelines were revised in 2000 to reflect current scientific knowledge on diet and health.

The ten guidelines are grouped under three messages that represent the ABC's for good health: (1) Aim for fitness; (2) Build a healthy base; and (3) Choose sensibly.

Aim for Fitness

- Aim for a healthy weight.
- Be physically active each day.

Aim for a healthy weight. Individuals who are overweight or obese are at greater risk for high blood pressure, heart disease, stroke, diabetes, certain types of cancer, arthritis, and breathing problems. Individuals at a healthy weight should try to avoid gaining weight. Overweight individuals should first try to prevent further weight gain and then try to lose weight.

Individuals who are overweight can improve their health, ability to function, and quality of life by losing 5–15% of their body weight. Six months is a reasonable period of time to lose 10% of body weight. A gradual weight loss of one-half to two pounds per week is recommended. Effective weight management requires increased physical activity and decreased consumption of calories over the long-term.

The Guidelines also recommend measuring around the waist, since excess fat in the abdomen (rather than the hips or thighs) increases the risk of heart disease and diabetes. If the waist measurement is greater than 35 inches for a woman or 40 inches for a man, the individual probably has excess abdominal fat.

Healthy weight (based on body composition) for athletes and active people is discussed in Chapter 10.

Be physically active each day. Every American should accumulate 30 minutes or more of moderate physical activity on most, preferably all, days of the week. One way to meet this goal is by walking two miles in 30 minutes. The activity can be done all at once or spread out over two or three periods during the day. Individuals can choose activities that fit with their daily routine (walking the stairs, gardening, mowing the lawn) or choose recreational or structured exercise programs (dancing, jogging, basketball) or do both. Even greater health benefits can be achieved by increasing the intensity or duration of physical activity.

Build a Healthy Base

- Let the Pyramid guide your food choices.
- Choose a variety of grains daily, especially whole grains.
- Choose a variety of fruits and vegetables daily.
- Keep food safe to eat.

Let the Pyramid guide your food choices. Since different foods contain different nutrients and other healthy substances, individuals should use the Pyramid to make healthy, enjoyable food choices. Plant foods that are nutrient-dense (whole grains, fruits, and vegetables), nonfat or low-fat dairy products, and low-fat foods from the meat and beans group are the foundation of a healthy diet. It's fine to enjoy sweets and fats on occasion.

Choose a variety of grains daily, especially whole grains. The Guidelines recommend consuming six or more servings of grain products daily. Several of these servings should be whole-grain foods, such as whole wheat, brown rice, oats, and whole corn. Grain products that contain little added saturated fat and low amounts of added sugars should be emphasized.

Choose a variety of fruits and vegetables daily. The Guidelines recommend consuming at least two servings of fruits and three servings of vegetables each day. Dark-green leafy vegetables, bright-orange fruits and vegetables, and cooked dried beans and peas should be eaten often.

Keep food safe to eat. The Guidelines recommend washing hands and food preparation surfaces often. Raw, cooked, and ready-to-eat foods should be separated during storage and preparation. Foods should be cooked at a safe temperature, and perishable foods should be promptly refrigerated. When the safety of the food is in doubt, it should be thrown out.

Choose Sensibly

- Choose a diet that is low in saturated fat and cholesterol and moderate in total fat.
- Choose beverages and foods that limit your intake of sugars.
- Choose and prepare foods with less salt.
- If you drink alcoholic beverages, do so in moderation.

Choose a diet that is low in saturated fat and cholesterol and moderate in total fat. Aim for a total fat intake of 30% of total calories. Try to consume less than 10% of calories from saturated fat and less than 300 milligrams of cholesterol per day. For example, at 2,200 calories per day, the upper limit on total fat is 660 calories (73 grams) and the upper limit on saturated fat is 220 calories (24 grams). As shown by the sample food label (Figure 2-2), one serving of the food has 3 grams of fat.

FIGURE 2-2.
A Sample Food Label

Reading the label tells more about the food and what you are getting. What you see on the food label—the nutrition and ingredient information—is required by the government. This shows what the new label looks like and explains some of its new features.

NUTRITION FACTS TITLE → *The new title "Nutrition Facts" signals the new label.*

NEW LABEL INFORMATION *The new nutrient list covers those most important to your health. You may have seen this information on some old labels, but it is now required.*

VITAMINS AND MINERALS *Only two vitamins, A and C, and two minerals, calcium and iron, are required on the food label. A food company can voluntarily list other vitamins and minerals in the food.*

LABEL NUMBERS *Numbers on the nutrition label may be rounded for labeling.*

Nutrition Facts

Serving Size 1 cup (228g) ◄
Servings Per Container: 2

Amount Per Serving

Calories 90	Calories from Fat 30

	% Daily Value*
Total Fat 3g	5%
Saturated Fat 0g	0%
Cholesterol 0 mg	0%
Sodium 300 mg	13%
Total Carbohydrate 13g	4%
Dietary Fiber 3g	12%
Sugars 3g	
Protein 3g	

Vitamin A 80%	•	Vitamin C 60%
Calcium 4%	•	Iron 4%

*Percent Daily Values are based on a 2,000 calorie diet. Your daily values may be higher or lower depending on your calorie needs:

	Calories	2,000	2,500
Total Fat	Less than	65g	80g
Sat Fat	Less than	20g	25g
Cholesterol	Less than	300mg	300mg
Sodium	Less than	2,400mg	2,400mg
Total Carbohydrate		300g	375g
Dietary Fiber		265g	30g

Calories per gram:

Fat 9 • Carbohydrate 4 • Protein 4

SERVING SIZE *Similar food products now have similar serving sizes. This makes it easier to compare foods. Serving sizes are based on amounts people actually eat.*

% DAILY VALUE *shows how a food fits into a 2,000 calorie reference diet. You can use % Daily Value to compare foods and see how the amount of a nutrient in a serving of food fills in a 2,000 calorie reference diet.*

DAILY VALUES FOOTNOTE *Daily Values are the new label reference numbers. These numbers are set by the government and are based on current nutrition recommendations.*

Some labels list the daily values for a daily diet of 2,000 and 2,500 calories. Your own nutrient needs may be less than or more than the Daily Values on the label.

The Guidelines recommend consuming two to three daily servings of fat-free or low-fat dairy products and two to three daily servings of cooked dried beans and peas, fish and lean meats, and poultry. Vegetable oils should be chosen rather than solid fats (meat and dairy fats, hard margarine, and shortening).

Choose beverages and foods that limit your intake of sugars. Sugars can promote tooth decay. The Guidelines recommend brushing and flossing teeth regularly and using fluoride toothpaste. Sugar and sugar-rich sweets are high in calories and low in nutrients, and they can crowd out nutrient-rich foods needed to maintain health.

Choose and prepare foods with less salt. Sodium, which is primarily supplied by salt, plays an essential role in regulating fluids and blood pressure. A teaspoon of table salt (sodium chloride) provides 2,400 milligrams of sodium. A high sodium intake is associated with higher blood pressure. The Guidelines recommend using herbs, spices, and fruits to flavor food and decreasing the amount of salty seasonings. The sodium needs of active people are discussed in Chapter 9.

If you drink alcoholic beverages, do so in moderation. Excessive alcohol consumption can increase the risk for automobile and other accidents, high blood pressure, stroke, violence, suicide, birth defects, and certain cancers. Too much alcohol may also cause social and psychological problems, cirrhosis of the liver, inflammation of the pancreas, and damage to the brain and heart.

The Guidelines recommend no more than two drinks per day for men and one drink per day for women, preferably consumed with meals to slow absorption. One drink is considered to be 12 ounces of beer, 5 ounces of wine, or 1½ ounces of 80 proof liquor. Alcohol should be avoided before driving and other risky situations. Alcohol is practically devoid of nutrients and can increase the risk of malnutrition by displacing nutritious foods in the diet.

DEVELOPING A HIGH-CARBOHYDRATE DIET

Depending on the intensity and duration of your sport or activity, you should be consuming 6 to 10 grams of carbohydrate per kilogram of body weight daily. The carbohydrate needs of specific sports and activities are discussed in Chapters 4 and 5.

A practical high-carbohydrate diet can be created by using the **food exchange system.** The exchange lists are the basis of a meal-planning system developed by the American Dietetic Association and the American Diabetes Association.

There are six food-planning exchange lists: grain, vegetables, fruit, meat, milk, and fat (Table 2-3). Each lists foods that have about the same amount of carbohydrate, protein, fat, and calories. Any food on a list can be exchanged or traded for any other food on the same list.

These food exchange lists can be used to plan diets from 1,500 to 4,000 calories a day (Table 2-4). These diets supply about 60% carbohydrate, 15% protein, and less than 25% fat. The grain, fruit, and vegetable exchanges are emphasized because they're high in carbohydrate and low in fat. Foods from the milk list are also good sources of carbohydrate. Choose low-fat or nonfat foods from the milk and meat lists to keep your intake of fat low.

Sugary foods such as cookies, cake, pie, soft drinks, and candy can supply additional carbohydrate but are low in most other nutrients. While there's no harm in eating some high-carbohydrate "empty calories" once you've met your nutrient needs, you can't go wrong adding extra servings of nutrient-dense carbohydrates.

NUTRITION COUNSELING

Beware of self-proclaimed nutrition "experts" who recommend supplements and rigid diets. The title "nutritionist" can be used by anyone, regardless of training. Under the heading "nutritionist,"

TABLE 2-3
Food Group Exchanges

STARCH/BREAD/GRAINS
(80 calories)

15 grams carbohydrate
3 grams protein
0 grams fat

½ cup pasta, barley, cooked cereal
⅓ cup rice or dried cooked peas/beans
½ cup corn, peas, winter squash
1 small (3 oz) baked potato
4–6 crackers
1 slice bread or 6-inch tortilla
½ bagel, English muffin, pita
¾ cup dry flaked cereal
3 cups popcorn, no oil or butter
¾ oz pretzels

MEAT AND MEAT ALTERNATIVES
(55–100 calories)

0 grams carbohydrate
7 grams protein
3–8 grams fat

1 oz poultry, fish, beef, pork, lamb, etc.
1/4 cup tuna, salmon, cottage cheese
2 tbsp. peanut butter
1 egg
1 oz cheese
tofu (2½ inch x 2¾ inch x 1 inch)

VEGETABLES
(25 calories)

5 grams carbohydrate
2 grams protein
0 grams fat

½ cup cooked vegetables
1 cup raw vegetables
½ cup tomato or vegetable juice

MILK
(90–150 calories)

12 grams carbohydrate
8 grams protein
0–5 grams fat

1 cup milk: nonfat, low-fat, 1%,
    whole
1 cup yogurt: nonfat, low-fat, 1%,
    whole

FRUIT
(60 calories)

15 grams carbohydrate
0 grams protein
0 grams fat

1 medium fresh fruit
1 cup berries or melon
½ cup canned fruit (without sugar)
½ cup fruit juice
¼ cup dried fruit

FAT
(45 calories)

0 grams carbohydrate
0 grams protein
5 grams fat

1 tsp. margarine, oil, butter,
    mayonnaise
2 tsp. diet margarine, diet mayonnaise
1 tbsp. salad dressing, cream cheese,
    cream, nuts
2 tbsp. diet salad dressing, sour cream
1 slice bacon

TABLE 2-4
Training Diet Meal Plans

FOOD GROUP	NUMBER OF EXCHANGES PER CALORIE LEVEL					
	1,500	2,000	2,500	3,000	3,500	4,000
Milk	3	3	4	4	4	4
Meat	5	5	5	5	6	6
Fruit	5	6	7	9	10	12
Vegetable	3	3	3	5	6	7
Grain	7	11	16	18	20	24
Fat	2	3	5	6	8	10

you have more than a 50% chance of finding a person who has phony credentials or delivers inaccurate information. If you want individual nutrition counseling, consult a registered dietitian (credentials abbreviated R.D.).

A registered dietitian is a health-care professional who is educated in nutrition and food science. For a person to become an R.D., the American Dietetic Association (ADA) requires specific course work from an accredited university (minimum of a bachelor of science degree), completion of a nutrition internship at an approved hospital, and the passing of a national certification exam. Registered dietitians are required to continue their professional education by attending scientific meetings or by writing scientific papers and giving lectures to colleagues.

You can find an R.D. by requesting a referral from your physician or by contacting the nutrition department of a hospital, clinic, or community health agency. You can also check in the phone book under dietitians, nutritionists, and weight control—remember to look for the R.D. after the name.

There are registered dietitians who specialize in sports nutrition. They usually belong to the Sports, Cardiovascular, and Wellness Nutrition Group (abbreviated SCAN) of the ADA. You can be referred to SCAN members in your geographic area by calling the American Dietetic Association at 1-800-366-1655.

3

ENERGY
SYSTEMS
FOR EXERCISE

Your body must be continuously supplied with energy to perform its many complex functions. When you exercise, your body requires more energy. There must be a way to provide this additional energy or you would stop moving.

This chapter describes the body's energy systems and how food provides energy for exercise. It also discusses the factors that determine the type of fuel your muscles use during exercise. After reviewing exercise fuel usage, you'll have a better appreciation for the importance of carbohydrate in your diet.

ATP—THE ENERGY CURRENCY

The energy-rich chemical compound **adenosine triphosphate**, or simply **ATP**, is used for all energy-requiring processes within the cell. The energy released from the breakdown of ATP is used to power all body functions, such as muscle contraction, so ATP is considered the "energy currency" of the cell. Another energy-rich compound called **creatine phosphate**, or **CP**, provides a small reserve of quick energy. The energy released from the breakdown of ATP and CP stores sustains all-out exercise (such as sprinting 100 meters) for about 6 to 8 seconds.

ATP must be continuously produced to provide a steady supply of energy. The muscle cell produces and maintains ongoing stores of ATP, utilizing glucose from carbohydrates, fatty acids from fats, and, to a small extent, amino acids from proteins. The body extracts the energy from dietary or body stores of carbohydrate, fat, and protein to rebuild the energy-rich ATP.

ENERGY PRODUCTION

Chains of chemical reactions use food, oxygen, and water to supply energy at rest and during exercise. This is referred to as **metabolism**. ATP is produced continuously within muscle cells through two important energy systems. The **anaerobic**, or **lactic-acid**, energy system doesn't require oxygen and provides immediate energy. It soon needs help, however, from the **aerobic** energy system, which depends on a steady supply of oxygen.

For a limited period of time (about a minute), you can rely on the anaerobic energy system. The anaerobic system supplies most of the energy for an all-out 400-meter sprint. It allows you to briefly exercise at a level that exceeds your ability to provide oxygen to your muscles.

When you exercise beyond several minutes, such as running a mile, your body needs a continuous supply of oxygen. The aerobic energy system provides almost all of your energy during exercise that lasts four minutes or longer.

Anaerobic System

Glucose is the only fuel that can be used when oxygen is not available. Glucose is stored in the muscles and liver as glycogen—which is a long chain of glucose molecules hooked together. In the anaerobic energy system, glucose is broken down to a substance called pyruvate. When oxygen is not available, pyruvate is converted into lactic acid, forming two molecules of ATP.

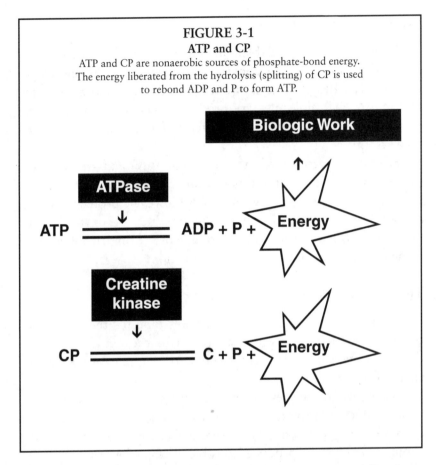

FIGURE 3-1
ATP and CP
ATP and CP are nonaerobic sources of phosphate-bond energy.
The energy liberated from the hydrolysis (splitting) of CP is used
to rebond ADP and P to form ATP.

Although the anaerobic system provides energy rapidly, there is a limit to the amount of lactic acid the body can tolerate. This is why anaerobic metabolism can fuel exercise for only a short period of time. When oxygen becomes available, lactic acid is converted back into pyruvate or burned directly by the muscles for energy. Lactic acid can also go to the liver and be converted back into glucose.

The anaerobic system provides energy for all-out effort lasting up to 60 seconds, such as sprinting and weight lifting. It also provides energy for bursts that are common in sports such as soccer, basketball, football, and tennis.

Aerobic System

When oxygen is available, glucose can be broken down more efficiently, without being converted to lactic acid. As shown in Figure 3-1, when glucose is broken down in the aerobic energy system, 36 ATP molecules are produced. This is 18 times more energy than when glucose is converted to lactic acid in the anaerobic system.

Fatty acids (from fat in the diet and body) and amino acids (from protein in the diet and body) can also go through the aerobic system to release energy as ATP. However, protein and fat cannot provide energy without the presence of oxygen. This means that when oxygen is limited, glucose (from carbohydrate) is the only fuel available for ATP production.

The Aerobic-Anaerobic Combination

At the beginning of exercise, it takes time for the heart and blood vessels to get oxygen-rich blood to the muscles. During this lag time, anaerobic ATP production supplies most of the energy for exercise.

After several minutes, oxygen becomes available and aerobic ATP production provides most of the energy needed to sustain exercise. However, when the exercise becomes too intense for enough energy to be produced aerobically (as when running up a hill or sprinting in a marathon), the body relies on the anaerobic system for more energy. This additional ATP is generated at the cost of increasing the lactic acid level in the blood.

In an event lasting several minutes, such as an 800-meter run, the contributions of aerobic and anaerobic ATP are about equal. As the distance (or time) increases, the contribution of aerobically produced energy increases (see Figure 3-2).

Although anaerobic energy production determines performance during sprint-type activities, the capacity to produce ATP aerobically determines endurance performance. Thus, the availability of oxygen in large part determines the potential for aerobic exercise.

FIGURE 3-2
The Anaerobic and Aerobic Reaction Systems Working Together

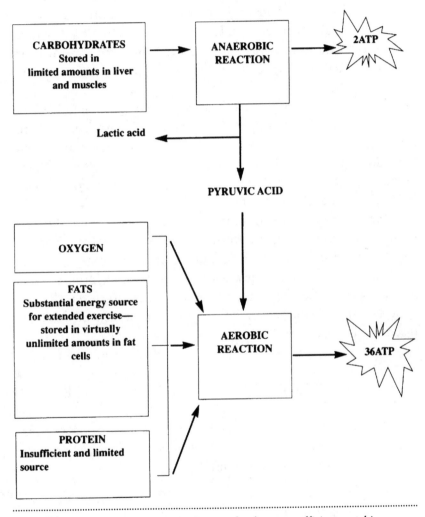

When enough oxygen is present in the muscle, the more efficient aerobic reaction system operates to provide the energy (ATP) used for muscle contractions. The aerobic system is very efficient and can produce up to 18 times the amount of ATP produced by the anaerobic system.

The aerobic system can utilize fats and, to a lesser extent, proteins, which are stored in virtually unlimited amounts in the body.

Your capacity for exercise intensity and duration are inversely related. That is, as the distance (or time) increases, you have to reduce your intensity, or pace. For example, a runner can't run a marathon (26.2 miles) as fast as a 10-kilometer race (6.2 miles). You can perform only at a certain percentage of your maximum aerobic capacity (abbreviated as VO_{2max}) for any given distance or time.

The aerobic energy system cannot tolerate the same level of intensity as the duration increases. Trained distance runners can run 1,500 meters, or a mile, at 100% of their aerobic capacity. In a 5-kilometer race (3.1 miles), they can use about 95% of their aerobic capacity. In a 10-kilometer race, they can average about 90% of their aerobic capacity.

During prolonged endurance exercise, there is an additional reason why you cannot perform close to your aerobic capacity for the entire distance. During endurance exercise that exceeds 90–120 minutes, muscle glycogen stores become progressively lowered. When this happens, you must either stop exercising or continue at a much slower pace. Muscle glycogen depletion is discussed in Chapters 4 and 5.

DETERMINANTS OF EXERCISE FUEL USAGE

A variety of factors determine which type of fuel your muscles will use during exercise. These include exercise intensity, exercise duration, and training level.

Intensity

The intensity of exercise is particularly important in determining your muscles' energy source. High-intensity, short-duration exercise (such as sprinting) relies on the anaerobic system for energy production. Only glucose, derived primarily from the breakdown of muscle glycogen, can be used as fuel.

FIGURE 3-3
The Anaerobic and Aerobic Continuum

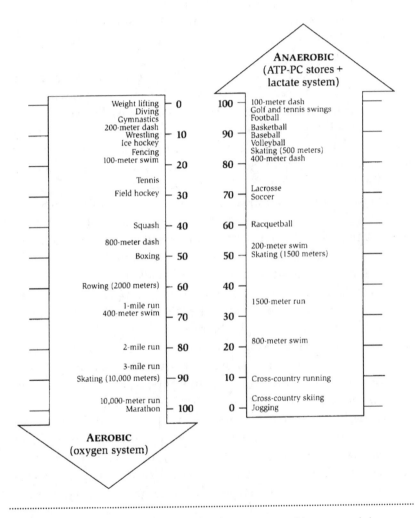

Whereas the 100-meter dash is considered a pure anaerobic event and the marathon a pure aerobic event, most other activities use ATP from both systems. Athletes should train both systems in accordance with the demands of their sport.

When glucose is broken down anaerobically, muscle glycogen is used 18 times faster than when glucose is broken down aerobically. A more rapid rate of muscle glycogen breakdown will also occur during high-intensity exercise (over 70% of aerobic capacity) when the anaerobic system is pulled in to assist the aerobic system in ATP production.

Extended mixed anaerobic-aerobic intermittent exercise like football drills, soccer, basketball, and running or swimming intervals also causes a greater breakdown of muscle glycogen.

Muscle glycogen and blood glucose supply half of the energy for aerobic exercise during a moderate workout (at or below 60% of aerobic capacity) and supply nearly all the energy during a hard workout (over 80% of aerobic capacity).

Exercise of low- to moderate-intensity (up to 60% of aerobic capacity) can be fueled almost entirely aerobically. The hormonal changes that occur with exercise—increased epinephrine (adrenaline) and decreased insulin levels—prompt muscle and fat (adipose) tissue to break down fat to fatty acids. Fatty acids derived from intramuscular fat and adipose tissue supply about half of the energy for low- to moderate-intensity exercise. Muscle glycogen and blood glucose supply the rest.

There are several reasons why fat cannot be used as fuel during high-intensity exercise (above 70% of aerobic capacity). First, the breakdown of fat to ATP is a slow process and cannot supply ATP fast enough to provide energy for high-intensity exercise.

Also, glucose provides more calories per liter of oxygen than does fat. Glucose delivers 5.10 calories per liter of oxygen, and fat delivers 4.62 calories per liter of oxygen. When less oxygen becomes available, as during high-intensity exercise, using glucose gives the muscles a distinct advantage because less oxygen is needed to produce energy.

Last, the shift in fuel from fat to glycogen as the exercise intensity increases is also partly due to the accumulation of lactic acid. During high-intensity exercise, lactic acid hinders the use of fat by the muscles. Thus, the muscles must rely more on glycogen for energy production.

Duration

The duration of exercise also defines whether the fuel used will be mostly muscle glycogen or fat. The longer you exercise, the greater the contribution of fat as fuel. Fat can supply as much as 60–70% of the energy needs for moderate-intensity exercise lasting 4 to 6 hours.

As the duration of exercise increases, the intensity must decrease, since there is a limited supply of stored glycogen. When muscle glycogen stores are low, fat breakdown supplies most of the energy needed for exercise. However, fat can be used as fuel only up to 60% of aerobic capacity. Also, a certain level of carbohydrate breakdown is necessary for fat to be burned for energy. To this extent, "fat burns in a carbohydrate flame."

As a result of the relationship between exercise intensity and duration, muscle glycogen is the predominant fuel for most types of exercise. It takes at least 20 minutes for fat to be available to the muscles as fuel in the form of free fatty acids. Most people don't train long enough to burn significant amounts of fat during the exercise session itself. Also, most people train and compete at an exercise intensity of 70% of aerobic capacity or above, which limits the use of fat as fuel.

This does not mean that you have to work out for a long time to lose body fat. When your workout creates a calorie deficit, the body will pull from its fat stores at a later time to make up that deficit. We discuss the benefits of exercise for body fat loss in Chapters 7 and 11.

Because fat is an important fuel source during prolonged exercise, some endurance athletes think they should eat a high-fat diet. This isn't necessary, since even the leanest athletes have more fat stored than they will ever use during exercise. The goal is to increase the utilization of fat as fuel through endurance training. Also, as Chapter 7 points out, a high-fat diet can increase your risk of health problems.

Keep in mind that eating too much fat also decreases carbohydrate intake. As Chapter 5 indicates, a low-carbohydrate diet lowers muscle glycogen stores. This decreases the body's ability to sustain high-intensity exercise and limits endurance. Thus, the ideal diet supplies enough carbohydrate (6 to 10 grams of carbohydrate per kilogram of body weight—about 55–65% carbohydrate) to ensure optimal muscle glycogen stores.

Training Level

Your training level will also determine what fuel your muscles use during exercise. Endurance (aerobic) training increases your aerobic capacity. This translates into greater fat utilization because a higher aerobic capacity increases your ability to perform more aerobically at the same absolute level of exercise.

The delivery of blood by the heart and the extraction of oxygen from the blood by the muscles determine your aerobic capacity. Ultimate aerobic capacity seems to be genetically determined, but whether or not you reach your full potential depends on training.

Endurance training also increases the threshold at which lactic acid starts to accumulate in the blood. Untrained people have a **lactate threshold** at about 50% of aerobic capacity. Trained people have a lactate threshold at about 70% of aerobic capacity. Lactic acid speeds up the rate of muscle glycogen breakdown by interfering with the use of fat as fuel. A higher lactate threshold enables you to use more fat and less glycogen at the same absolute level of exercise.

Endurance training also causes several major adaptations in the muscles that promote greater fat utilization. Endurance training increases the amount and activity of the specific muscle enzymes that are responsible for burning fat. It also increases the number of capillaries in the trained muscles so that the muscles receive more blood and oxygen. When more fat is burned, less glycogen is used. This "glycogen sparing" effect is beneficial because muscle glycogen stores are limited and fat stores are abundant.

Lastly, endurance training increases the capacity of the muscles to store glycogen. Thus, endurance training confers a dual performance advantage: Muscle glycogen stores are higher at the onset of exercise, and they are used up at a slower rate.

4

EATING
FOR YOUR
SPORT

M any athletes are confused about what to eat before and during training and competition. This chapter provides recommendations for fueling before and during exercise based on the duration of your sport. Nutrition guidelines to enhance recovery are discussed in the next chapter.

Eating well during training is just as important as eating well for competition. Proper dietary habits help you to train harder so that you're better prepared for competition.

EATING BEFORE EXERCISE

Many athletes train and compete in the morning without eating. This overnight fast lowers liver glycogen stores—the body's main source of blood glucose. Eating a high-carbohydrate meal before morning exercise will help to maintain blood glucose levels so that you can perform at your best.

During exercise, athletes rely primarily on their pre-existing muscle glycogen and fat stores. Although the pre-exercise meal doesn't contribute immediate energy, it can provide energy when exercising longer than an hour. The carbohydrate in the meal raises blood glucose to provide energy for the working muscles. The pre-exercise meal also helps prevent feelings of hunger and weakness, which can harm performance.

Consume your carbohydrate-rich meal one to four hours before training or competition. This allows adequate time for food to empty from the stomach. Exercising with a nearly full stomach can cause indigestion, nausea, and vomiting as blood is diverted from the stomach to the muscles.

The amount to consume depends on the timing of the meal. To avoid potential gastrointestinal distress, the carbohydrate and calorie content of the meal should be reduced the closer to exercise the meal is consumed. For example, a small meal of 300 to 400 calories is appropriate an hour before exercise, whereas a large meal of 700 to 800 calories can be consumed four hours before exercise.

Good examples of high-carbohydrate foods for pre-exercise meals include bread products such as toast, bagels, pancakes, or muffins (adding jam or jelly increases the carbohydrate content), cooked or dry cereal, fruit, sports bars, nonfat or 1% fat yogurt, and liquid meals. Fruit juices, nonfat or 1% fat milk, and sports drinks are good high-carbohydrate beverages. Table 4-1 provides examples of pre-exercise meals.

Fatty foods should be limited because fat slows stomach emptying time and may make you feel sluggish and heavy. Many popular high-protein breakfast foods (bacon, sausage, and cheese) are high in fat. In contrast, carbohydrates provide the quickest and most efficient source of energy and, unlike fats, are rapidly digested.

You may need to watch your fiber intake (especially bran) in your pre-exercise meal to avoid abdominal cramping and a bathroom break during exercise. This is merely annoying during training, but can be disastrous during competition. It's also a good idea to minimize gas-forming foods such as beans and onions. Extremely salty foods (bacon and sausage) can cause fluid retention and a bloated feeling. Above all, you should choose palatable, familiar, and well-tolerated foods.

TABLE 4-1
Examples of Pre-event Meals

BREAKFAST
Orange juice
Blueberry pancakes with syrup
Bagel
Low-fat yogurt
Banana

Cranberry juice
Cornflakes
Low-fat milk
Apple muffin

....

LUNCH/DINNER
Chicken sandwich on whole-wheat roll
Fruit cup
Fig bar
Frozen low-fat yogurt

Low-fat milk
Pasta with tomato sauce
Salad with tomato, carrots, cucumbers, and mushrooms
Italian bread
Fresh fruit
Low-fat milk
Sherbet

Baked potato with low-fat cheese
Cornmeal muffin
Low-fat vanilla milk shake

Thick crust cheese and mushroom pizza
Low-fat milk
Fresh fruit
Bread sticks

✓ Note: Caloric intake depends on length of time before event.

Experimenting with a variety of pre-exercise meals in training helps determine what foods are most likely to settle well before competition. Many people are tense before competing, which slows down digestion. Even familiar, well-tolerated foods may take longer to digest. Never try an untested food or fluid before competition. The result may be severe indigestion and impaired performance.

Drinking fluids with your pre-exercise meal and before exercise helps to ensure that you're properly hydrated. Caffeine-containing beverages such as coffee, tea, and soda may cause problems for some individuals, particularly young athletes. The side effects of consuming caffeine—agitation, nausea, muscle tremors, palpitations, and headache—can impair performance.

Caffeine is also a diuretic. An excessive intake of caffeine can stimulate the production of urine and cause water losses. Caffeine's diuretic effect may contribute to dehydration and reduced endurance in hot weather if you don't hydrate properly. Hydration guidelines and appropriate fluid-replacement beverages are discussed in Chapter 9.

Some athletes have "lucky" foods they associate with peak performance. As long as these foods don't cause indigestion or hinder performance, it's fine to include them even if they don't meet the recommendations for pre-exercise meals.

Liquid Meals

A number of commercially formulated liquid meals are available, as shown in Table 4-2. Their fluid and carbohydrate content makes them a desirable meal choice either before competition or during day-long competitions such as swim meets, track meets, tennis tournaments, volleyball, and wrestling. Liquid meals can also be used for nutritional supplementation during heavy training when you need a lot of calories.

Liquid meals have several advantages over conventional meals. They leave the stomach more rapidly than regular meals, thereby helping to prevent nausea before competition. Liquid

TABLE 4-2
Nutrition Beverages

Beverage	Flavors	Calories per 8-oz. serving	Carbohydrate (Grams)	Protein (Grams)	Fat (Grams)
GatorPro® Sports Nutritiont Supplement GATORADE COMPANY	Chocolate, vanilla	360	58	16	7
Sport Shake MID-AMERICA FARMS	Chocolate, vanilla, strawberry	310	45	11	10
Endura Optimizer® UNIPRO, INC.	Chocolate vanilla, orange	260	57	11	less than 1
Protein Repair Formula® PUREPOWER SPORTS NUTRITION	Vanilla	200	26	20	1.5
Metabolol II® CHAMPION NUTRITION	Plain	260	40	20	2
Ensure ROSS LABORATORIES	Chocolate, Strawberry, Vanilla	254	35	9	9
Nutrament® MEAD JOHNSON NUTRITIONALS	Chocolate, banana, vanilla, strawberry, coconut	240	34	6.5	11
Sustacal® MEAD JOHNSON NUTRITIONALS	Chocolate, vanilla, strawberry, eggnog	240	33	5.5	14.5
Go!	Vanilla, chocolate, strawberry, banana, orange cream	235	40	14	3

meals also produce a low stool residue. This helps to keep immediate weight gain to a minimum and decreases the risk of a bathroom break during exercise.

Liquid meals satisfy hunger and supply energy without giving an uncomfortable feeling of fullness. Many athletes value a feeling of "lightness," especially as they enter competition.

You can concoct homemade liquid meals by mixing 1% fat milk, fruit, and nonfat dry milk powder in a blender. For variety, add cereal, yogurt, and flavoring (vanilla and chocolate). You can also use sugar and honey for additional sweetness and carbohydrate. There are several brands of "instant breakfast" powders that can be mixed with milk.

EATING FOR SHORT-DURATION EVENTS

There are several important steps to get ready for an all-out event lasting up to four minutes. First, the muscles' stores of ATP, CP, and glycogen shouldn't be exhausted by hard exercise immediately before the event. Also, your calorie intake should be adequate for several days prior to the event. During training, you should eat at least the minimum number of servings from the Food Guide Pyramid.

Athletes are often involved in several events during track and swim meets. Though each event may not last long, the repeated bursts of all-out effort may significantly reduce muscle glycogen stores. If possible, enough time should be allowed between events to restore muscle glycogen to optimal levels.

Recovery periods are also necessary to clear the muscles of the buildup of lactic acid from anaerobic metabolism. Muscle glycogen depletion from repetitive events and the accumulation of lactic acid can both impair your performance.

Athletes in short-term events require fluids and carbohydrate throughout the day of the meet. Some people may be reluctant to eat and drink because they have to compete again.

However, failing to refuel and replace fluid losses can cause performance to deteriorate, particularly toward the end of the day. Since everything eaten before an event may be considered a preevent meal, it's important to consider the amount of time between competitions.

If there is less than an hour between competitions, you can drink sports drinks, water, and fruit juices. When there are several hours between events, eat easily digestible carbohydrate-rich foods such as fruit, grain products (fig bars, bagels, graham crackers), low-fat yogurt, sports bars, and liquid meals in addition to drinking fluids. When your events are separated by three hours or more, you can consume high-carbohydrate meals along with drinking fluids.

Carbohydrate feedings can also improve performance in stop-and-go sports such as basketball, football, volleyball, and soccer that require repeated bouts of high-intensity, short-duration effort.

EATING FOR INTERMEDIATE-LENGTH EVENTS

A variety of sports require intense exertion for periods of 4 to 10 minutes and longer. The mile run, wrestling matches, middle-distance swimming events, and rowing contests all demand maximal effort without rest.

Since muscle glycogen is the predominant fuel for these events, athletes must ensure that their muscle glycogen stores are adequate when they enter competition. While the events themselves usually aren't long enough to cause muscle glycogen depletion, heavy training in preparation for competition can significantly lower muscle glycogen stores. If muscle glycogen stores haven't been replenished prior to competition (restoration of muscle glycogen takes 24 to 48 hours), performance will suffer. To guarantee optimal muscle glycogen stores, you should taper training several days prior to competition and eat a high-carbohydrate diet.

Athletes in intermediate events must also be well-hydrated to perform at their best. Some people don't adequately replace their fluid losses between training sessions and are dehydrated when they enter competition. Dehydration impairs performance and increases the risk of heat illnesses.

EATING FOR ENDURANCE EVENTS

Training for and competing in endurance events such as cross-country running and skiing, triathlons, and bicycle road-racing significantly lowers muscle and liver glycogen stores. Muscle glycogen depletion is a well-recognized limitation to endurance performance. Athletes who train exhaustively on successive days must consume adequate carbohydrate and calories to prevent the cumulative depletion of muscle glycogen.

Endurance athletes should consume a carbohydrate-rich meal one to four hours before prolonged training and competition. Consuming carbohydrate during events lasting an hour or longer also improves endurance by providing glucose for the muscles to use when their glycogen stores have dropped to low levels.

Endurance athletes who compete for longer than 90 minutes can improve their performance by maximizing their muscle glycogen stores in the week prior to the event. This dietary program, called carbohydrate loading, is discussed in the next chapter.

Proper hydration is the most important nutritional concern during prolonged endurance exercise. An endurance athlete can collapse from heat exhaustion or heatstroke long before muscle glycogen stores are depleted. Endurance athletes in particular are susceptible to impaired performance from chronic dehydration. Fluid-replacement guidelines and beverages are discussed in Chapter 9.

REFUELING DURING EXERCISE

Taking in carbohydrate-rich foods and fluids during stop-and-go and endurance sports lasting an hour or longer can improve performance. Consuming carbohydrate provides glucose for muscles when they're running low on glycogen. This enables the production of energy to continue at a high rate and your performance is enhanced. In practical terms, you can maintain your pace longer and/or sprint harder at the end of exercise.

The liver supplies glucose to maintain blood glucose level. As muscles run out of glycogen, they take up more blood glucose, placing a drain on the liver glycogen stores. The longer the exercise session, the greater the utilization of blood glucose for energy. When the liver glycogen is depleted, blood glucose drops. While a few people may experience symptoms of low blood sugar such as dizziness, most have to reduce their exercise intensity because of muscle fatigue.

Try to consume 30 to 60 grams of carbohydrate (120 to 240 calories) every hour. You can obtain this amount from either carbohydrate-rich foods (such as sports bars, gels, fig bars, fruit, and cookies) and/or sports drinks.

Each carbohydrate form (liquid versus solid) has advantages and drawbacks. High-carbohydrate foods can be easily carried and provide a feeling of satiety that you won't get from drinking fluids. Sports bars, fig bars, and cookies have a very low water content, so are more compact. By comparison, high-carbohydrate foods that have a high water content, such as fruit, take up more room. For example, to get the amount of carbohydrate supplied by one PowerBar (47 grams), you'd have to eat 1½ bananas (45 grams).

However, the low water content of some high-carbohydrate solid foods also has a downside. You'd better drink plenty of water when you eat solid food, especially a sports bar. Otherwise, the food can settle poorly and you may feel like there's a rock in your gut. In addition to aiding your digestion, drinking water while eating solid foods encourages you to hydrate adequately.

Eating one banana (30 grams of carbohydrate), one Power Bar (47 grams of carbohydrate), two gels (about 50 grams of carbohydrate), four small fig bars (42 grams of carbohydrate), or two large graham crackers (42 grams of carbohydrate) every hour supplies an adequate amount of carbohydrate.

Sports drinks are a practical source of carbohydrate because they also replace fluid losses. They provide the right proportion of water to carbohydrate to provide energy quickly and replace fluid losses. Drinking 20 to 40 ounces of a properly formulated sports drink (4–8% carbohydrate) each hour also provides the proper amount of carbohydrate. For example, drinking 20 ounces of Gatorade every hour provides 36 grams of carbohydrate.

Try to eat and drink before feeling hungry or tired, usually within 30 minutes after starting to exercise. Consuming small amounts at frequent intervals (every 30 to 60 minutes) helps to promote hydration, maintain blood glucose levels, and prevent gastrointestinal upset. Your foods and fluids should be easily digestible, familiar (tested in training), and enjoyable (to encourage eating and drinking).

5

CARBOHYDRATES: YOUR HIGH-OCTANE FUEL

Muscle glycogen represents the major source of carbohydrate in the body (300 to 400 grams or 1,200 to 1,600 calories), followed by liver glycogen (75 to 100 grams or 300 to 400 calories) and, lastly, blood glucose (25 grams or 100 calories).

Muscle glycogen is the preferred fuel for most types of exercise. Replenishing and maintaining glycogen stores during training and prior to competition requires a carbohydrate-rich diet. This chapter reviews carbohydrate requirements for training and the role of nutrient-dense carbohydrates and sugar in the diet. The benefits of consuming carbohydrate for recovery and carbohydrate loading are also discussed.

CARBOHYDRATE NEEDS FOR TRAINING

Have you ever had days of training when you felt that you'd lost speed, precision, and endurance? Many such bad days are caused by low levels of glycogen in your muscles.

Glycogen depletion can occur gradually over repeated days of heavy training when glycogen breakdown exceeds its replacement.

45

When this happens, glycogen stores drop lower with each successive day and workouts become more difficult and less enjoyable. The deterioration in performance and feeling of sluggishness associated with glycogen depletion is often referred to as "staleness" and blamed on overtraining.

Glycogen depletion can occur while training for sports that require repeated, near-maximal bursts of effort (such as basketball, soccer, and football) as well as during endurance sports. Glycogen depletion is often accompanied by a sudden weight loss of several pounds (due to glycogen and water loss) and you can't maintain your usual training intensity. When you don't consume enough carbohydrate or calories and/or don't take days off to rest, you're a prime candidate for glycogen depletion. Most Americans consume only 49% carbohydrate or about 5 grams of carbohydrate per kilogram of body weight daily. (One kilogram equals 2.2 pounds.)

You can prevent glycogen depletion by consuming a carbohydrate-rich diet (6 to 10 grams of carbohydrate per kilogram daily) and taking periodic rest days to give your muscles time to rebuild their stores. You should consume at least 6 grams of carbohydrate per kilogram daily (about 55% of your total calories) if you're working out for an hour each day. A diet containing 8 to 10 grams of carbohydrate per kilogram is recommended when you're training hard for several hours or more each day. As we'll discuss later in this chapter, a high-carbohydrate diet is even more critical for recovery from prolonged, heavy exercise.

As an example, a 154-pound (70-kilogram) person who trains strenuously for an hour needs 420 grams of carbohydrate daily. You can determine the carbohydrate content of different foods by reading food labels. Table 5-1 gives some examples of high-carbohydrate foods. You can also use the food exchange lists (Chapter 2) to develop a high-carbohydrate diet.

As a general guide, starchy foods and fruits provide the highest amount of carbohydrate (15 grams) per serving. A serving of starch consists of 1 slice of bread or small tortilla, ½ cup pasta or cooked cereal, ⅓ cup cooked rice or beans, or 1 small potato. A serving of fruit is 1 medium-size fruit, 1 cup berries or melon, ½ cup juice, or ¼ cup dried fruit.

Milk is the next highest source, providing 12 grams of carbohydrate for 1 cup of milk or yogurt (choose nonfat or 1% fat products to keep fat intake down). Vegetables provide 5 grams of carbohydrate per ½ cup cooked vegetables, 1 cup raw vegetables, or ½ cup tomato or vegetable juice.

THE ROLE OF SUGAR AND SUGAR MYTHS

Sugary foods such as cakes, cookies, pies, soft drinks, and candy can help increase carbohydrate and calorie intake during training. However, these foods should be eaten in addition to, not in place of, nutrient-dense carbohydrate foods. When sugar replaces complex carbohydrates in the diet, intake of vitamins, minerals, and fiber will be reduced. Many sugary baked goods and candy are also high in fat.

Despite popular press claims, brown sugar, date sugar, honey, and molasses are not nutritionally superior to table sugar. Although they do contain trace amounts of some vitamins and minerals, consuming these so-called natural sugars will not add significant nutritional value to your diet.

Some athletes think that fructose is a better energy source than other sugars because fructose causes a lower insulin response than glucose. However, consuming fructose does not improve endurance and has even been shown to harm performance. You store twice as much muscle glycogen after eating glucose or sucrose compared to eating fructose. Also, fructose is far more likely to cause gastrointestinal distress, even in small amounts. For this reason, glucose, maltodextrins (glucose polymers), and sucrose are the major carbohydrate sources in sports drinks. Maltodextrins are created by breaking down cornstarch into small glucose chains (polymers).

TABLE 5-1
High-Carbohydrate Foods

FOOD GROUP	CALORIES	CARBOHYDRATES (GRAMS)
Milk		
Low-fat (2%) milk (1 cup)	121	12
Skim milk (1 cup)	86	12
Chocolate milk (1 cup)	208	26
Pudding, any flavor (½ cup)	161	30
Frozen yogurt, low-fat (1 cup)	220	34
Fruit-flavored low-fat yogurt (1 cup)	225	42
Beans		
Blackeye peas (½ cup)	134	22
Pinto beans (1 cup)	235	44
Navy beans (1 cup)	259	48
Refried beans (½ cup)	142	26
Garbanzo beans (chickpeas) (1 cup)	269	45
White beans (1 cup)	249	45
Fruits		
Apple (1 medium)	81	21
Apple juice (1 cup)	111	28
Applesauce (1 cup)	232	60
Banana (1)	105	27
Canteloupe (1 cup)	57	14
Dates, dried (10)	228	61
Fruit Roll-Ups (1 roll)	50	12
Grapes (1 cup)	114	28
Grape juice (1 cup)	96	23
Orange (1)	65	16
Orange juice (1 cup)	112	26
Pear (1)	98	25
Pineapple (1 cup)	77	19
Prunes, dried (10)	201	53
Raisins (⅔ cup)	302	79
Raspberries (1 cup)	61	14
Strawberries (1 cup)	45	11
Watermelon (1 cup)	50	12
Vegetables		
Three-bean salad (½ cup)	90	20
Carrots (1 medium)	31	8
Corn (½ cup)	89	21
Lima beans (½ cup)	108	20

TABLE 5-1 (continued)
High-Carbohydrate Foods

FOOD GROUP	CALORIES	CARBOHYDRATES (GRAMS)
Vegetables		
Peas, green (½ cup)	63	12
Potato (1 large)	220	50
Sweet Potato (1 large)	118	28
Grains		
Bagel (1)	165	31
Biscuit (1)	103	13
White bread (1 slice)	61	12
Whole-wheat bread (1 slice)	55	11
Breadsticks (2 sticks)	77	15
Cornbread (1 square)	178	28
Cereal, ready-to-eat (1 cup)	110	24
Oatmeal (½ cup)	66	12
Cream of Rice (¾ cup)	95	21
Cream of Wheat (¾ cup)	96	20
Flavored oatmeal, Quaker instant (1 packet)	110	25
Graham crackers (2 squares)	60	11
Saltines (5 crackers)	60	10
Triscuit crackers (3 crackers)	60	10
Pancake (4-inch diameter)	61	9
Waffles (2, 3.5" x 5.5")	130	17
Rice (1 cup)	223	50
Rice, brown (1 cup)	232	50
Hamburger bun (1)	119	21
Hotdog bun (1)	119	21
Noodles, spaghetti (1 cup)	159	34
Flour tortilla (1)	85	15
Oatmeal raisin cookie	62	9
Pizza (cheese, 1 slice)	290	39
Popcorn, plain (1 cup, popped)	26	6
English muffin	130	25
Fig bar (1)	50	10
Granola bar (honey and oats, 1 oz)	125	19
Pretzels (1 oz)	106	21

Consuming sugar before anaerobic exercise such as sprinting or weight lifting will not improve performance, because the body relies on stored ATP, CP, and muscle glycogen for these tasks. Sugar won't provide you with a sudden burst of quick energy, allowing you to exercise harder or longer. To the contrary, eating too much sugar immediately before or during exercise can increase the risk of gastrointestinal problems (cramps, nausea, diarrhea, and bloating).

THE ROLE OF NUTRIENT-DENSE CARBOHYDRATES

As discussed in Chapter 2, your primary food sources should be the whole-grain products, vegetables, and fruits at the bottom of the Food Guide Pyramid. These foods promote good health and athletic performance.

The dietary fiber found in whole grains, vegetables, and fruits may help reduce your risk of heart disease and certain cancers. The soluble fiber found in beans, oats, dried peas, and legumes can help to lower the cholesterol level in your blood. Since high blood cholesterol is a major risk factor for heart disease (see Chapter 7), consuming more soluble fiber may help reduce your risk for heart disease.

The insoluble fiber found in wheat bran, whole-grain products, and vegetables speeds up the movement of food through the gastrointestinal tract. Insoluble fiber may reduce your risk for bowel disorders such as diverticulitis and constipation. Fruits, barley, and vegetables are sources of both soluble and insoluble fiber. Table 5-2 lists the fiber content of selected foods.

In addition to fiber, minimally processed plant foods such as whole-grain products, vegetables, and fruits supply vitamins, minerals, and phytochemicals (plant chemicals) that have positive health effects. These foods are "nutrient dense"—they supply a significant amount of nutrients for their calories.

TABLE 5-2
Fiber Content of Foods

FOOD GROUP	SERVING SIZE	GRAMS OF DIETARY FIBER
Breads and Crackers		
Bran muffin	1 medium	3
Whole-wheat bread	1 slice	2
Oat bran, English muffin	1 muffin	3
Ry-Krisp	0.5 ounce	3
Crispbread, Wasa	1 piece	1–3
Cereals and Pasta		
General Mills Fiber One	1 ounce	13
Kellogg's All-Bran	1 ounce	10
Whole-wheat pasta	1 cup	5
Long-grain brown rice	1 cup	3
Kellogg's Bran Flakes	1 ounce	4
Oatmeal	1 cup	2
Popcorn	1 ounce	2
Fruits and Nuts		
Almonds	¼ cup	5
Dried prunes	3	4
Apple (with skin)	1 medium	3
Banana	1 medium	3
Dried dates	5	3
Nectarine	1 medium	3
Peach (with skin)	1 medium	3
Roasted peanuts	¼ cup	3
Strawberries	1 cup	3
Cantaloupe	¼ cup	2
Orange	1 medium	2
Smooth peanut butter	2 tbsp.	2
Walnut pieces	¼ cup	2
Pistachios	1 ounce	3
Cooked Legumes		
Kidney beans	½ cup	9
Baked beans	½ cup	7
Navy beans	½ cup	5
Pinto beans	½ cup	5
Lentils	½ cup	2

(continued on next page)

TABLE 5-2 (continued)
Fiber Content of Foods

FOOD GROUP	SERVING SIZE	GRAMS OF DIETARY FIBER
Vegetables		
Cooked frozen peas	½ cup	4
Baked potato (with skin)	1 medium	4
Cooked broccoli tops	½ cup	3
Cooked young carrots	½ cup	3
Cooked corn	½ cup	3
Cooked green beans	½ cup	2

Compare a small baked potato with a third of a candy bar, which both contain about 100 calories. The potato provides ample vitamin C, with a small amount of protein, B vitamins, about a half-dozen minerals, and fiber. The third of the candy bar provides the same amount of energy, about three times as much fat, and little or no fiber, vitamins, or minerals.

Contrary to popular belief, starches such as whole-grain breads and cereals, potatoes, corn, beans, rice, and pasta contribute significantly fewer calories for a given amount than foods with a high fat or sugar content. The "diet lunch" of a hamburger patty and a scoop of cottage cheese provides a lot of fat calories.

By replacing fats and sugary foods in the diet, nutrient-dense carbohydrates actually facilitate weight loss because they contain fewer calories. Also, the naturally occurring sugars in fruits make them ideal for a sweet, low-calorie treat.

COMMERCIAL CARBOHYDRATE SUPPLEMENTS

Some athletes train so heavily that they have difficulty eating enough food to meet their carbohydrate needs. This can happen for several reasons.

TABLE 5-3
Tips for Choosing Nutrient-Dense Foods

- Bring boundaries to your meals—watch portions of meals and snacks.
- Remember—nonfat does not mean calorie free!
- Choose nutrient-dense cereals such as Grapenuts, Total, Raisin Bran, and Wheat Chex. Top with bananas, strawberries, peaches, blueberries.
- Make oatmeal with nonfat milk rather than with water. Top with low-fat yogurt or fruit.
- Eat fruit instead of filling up on fruit juices between or with meals.
- Blend your own low-fat milk shakes or fruit smoothies for a meal or snack.
- Choose hearty, dense breads such as sprouted wheat, oat bran, and honey bran. Use thick slices for sandwiches and toast. Stuff with low-fat tuna salad, chicken salad, or veggies and low-fat cream cheese.
- Choose hearty soups such as minestrone, chicken and vegetable, black bean, or lentil.
- Bake or grill chicken, beef, or fish instead of frying. Use low-fat marinades, sauces, and herbs to add flavor in place of cream sauces or gravy.
- Include lower-calorie vegetables such as tomatoes, carrots, cucumbers, green and red peppers, broccoli, cauliflower, spinach, kale on a salad or as a snack.
- Try stir-fry chicken, lean beef, fish, or tofu with vegetables. Make hearty low-fat chili. Serve with brown or white rice.
- Use low-fat fajitas or wraps and add a combination of the following: veggies, chicken, low-fat ground turkey, nonfat refried beans, shrimp, low-fat cheese, nonfat sour cream, salsa, onions.
- Add low-fat cheese, low-fat cottage cheese, garbanzo beans, kidney beans, chopped eggs, and low-fat dressing to mixed-green salads.
- Try nutrient-dense snacks such as oatmeal raisin cookies, low-fat fig bars, low-fat puddings, low-fat frozen yogurt, low-fat fruit breads, low-fat crackers, low-fat granola bars, fruit.

The stress of hard training can decrease your appetite so that you don't consume enough calories and carbohydrate. Eating a large volume of food can also cause gastrointestinal discomfort and interfere with training. Some athletes spend so much time training that they don't have enough rest time available to replenish properly.

If you have problems consuming enough carbohydrate, you can use a commercial high-carbohydrate supplement. These products don't replace regular food but help supply additional calories and carbohydrate when needed.

You can use high-carbohydrate supplements before or after exercise, either with meals or between meals. They are too concentrated in carbohydrate (18–24%) to be used as fluid-replacement drinks during exercise.

CARBOHYDRATES AND RECOVERY

Replacing muscle glycogen stores following strenuous training is important to minimize chronic fatigue. Based on the time spent training, you should consume 6 to 10 grams of carbohydrate per kilogram each day (about 55–65% calories from carbohydrate).

It's also important to take in carbohydrate immediately (within 30 minutes) after hard workouts that last several hours. Consuming high-carbohydrate fluids and foods right after prolonged training and competitions increases glycogen storage and may help you recover faster. Replenishing muscle glycogen stores after exercise is particularly beneficial if you train hard several times a day. This will enable you to get the most out of your second workout.

Many people aren't hungry after heavy training. If you are not, consume a high-carbohydrate drink such as fruit juice or a commercial high-carbohydrate supplement. This will also promote rehydration.

TABLE 5-4
High-Carbohydrate Beverages

Beverage	Flavors	Carbohydrate Ingredient	Carbohydrate % (Concentration) 12-oz. Serving	Carbohydrate	Sodium
GatorLode® High-Carbohydrate Loading and Recovery Drink THE GATORADE COMPANY	Lemon, citrus, banana	Maltodextrin, glucose	20	70	95
Gatorade Torq THE GATORADE COMPANY	Wild berry, grape orange	Maltodextrin, glucose	21 21	77 77	0 0
Carboplex® UNIPRO, INC.	Plain	Maltodextrin	24	82	0
Carbo Power® NATURE'S BEST FOOD SUPPLEMENTS	Lemonade, strawberry, fruit punch, orange, grape, tea	Maltodextrin, high-fructose corn syrup	18	64	76
Ultra Fuel® TWIN LABS	Lemon, lime, grape, fruit punch, orange	Maltodextrin, glucose, fructose	21	75	0
ProOptibol® 105 NEXT NUTRITION	Wild berry	Glucose, fructose	19	66	0
Cybergenics Cybercharge® L & S RESEARCH CORP.	Lemon, lime, grape	Glucose, polymers, fructose	21	75	15
Carbo Fire® WEIDER HEALTH & FITNESS	Tropical punch, orange	Glucose, polymers, fructose	24	83	60

After hard workouts, try to consume 1.5 grams of carbohydrate per kilogram within 30 minutes of exercise, followed by an additional feeding of 1.5 gram per kilogram two hours later. The first carbohydrate feeding can be a high-carbohydrate beverage, and the second feeding can be a high-carbohydrate meal.

For example, a 70-kilogram man should consume 105 grams of carbohydrate within 30 minutes of exercise and two hours later. For the first feeding, he drinks 18 ounces of GatorLode. His second meal two hours later—two cups of spaghetti with ½ cup of tomato sauce and two pieces of french bread—provides 100 grams of carbohydrate.

CARBOHYDRATE LOADING

During endurance exercise that exceeds 90 to 120 minutes, such as running a marathon, muscle glycogen stores become progressively lower. When they drop to critically low levels (the point of glycogen depletion), you cannot maintain high-intensity exercise. In practical terms, you've "hit the wall" and must drastically reduce your pace.

Carbohydrate loading can increase muscle glycogen stores by 50–100%. The greater the pre-exercise muscle glycogen content, the greater the endurance potential. Table 5-3 gives an overview of the diet and training regimen used for carbohydrate loading.

On the sixth day before the event, you exercise hard (about 70% of aerobic capacity) for 90 minutes. On the fifth and fourth days before the event, decrease your training to 40 minutes. During the first three days, you consume a normal diet providing about 5 grams of carbohydrate per kilogram per day (about 50% carbohydrate). On the third and second days before the event, reduce your training to 20 minutes. On the day before the event, you rest. During the last three days, eat a high-carbohydrate diet providing 10 grams of carbohydrate per kilogram per day (about 65% carbohydrate).

TABLE 5-5
Training and Diet Regimen for Glycogen Loading

	TRAINING	EATING
DAY 1	90 min • 70-75% $\dot{V}O_{2max}$	50% Carbohydrate 5gm/kg
DAY 2	40 min • 70–75% $\dot{V}O_{2max}$	50% Carbohydrate 5gm/kg
DAY 3	40 min • 70–75% $\dot{V}O_{2\ max}$	50% Carbohydrate 5gm/kg
DAY 4	20 min • 70–75% $\dot{V}O_{2max}$	70% Carbohydrate 10gm/kg
DAY 5	20 min • 70–75% $\dot{V}Oxmax$	70% Carbohydrate 10gm/kg
DAY 6	Rest	70% Carbohydrate 10gm/kg
DAY 7	EVENT	EVENT

Endurance training is the primary stimulus for muscle glycogen synthesis. This means that you must be endurance trained or carbohydrate loading won't work. Also, the exercise to lower glycogen stores must be the same as your competitive event because glycogen stores are specific to the muscle groups used. For example, runners need to decrease their stores by running rather than cycling.

It's essential that you decrease your training the three days prior to competition. Too much exercise during this period will use too much stored glycogen and defeat the purpose of the whole process. The final three days, when you taper and eat a high-carbohydrate diet, is the real loading phase of the regimen.

If you have difficulty consuming enough carbohydrate from food, you can use a high-carbohydrate supplement. If you have heart disease, diabetes, and/or high blood triglycerides, you may have problems if you carbohydrate load. When in doubt, check with your doctor before attempting this regimen.

For each gram of glycogen stored, additional water is stored. Some people note a feeling of stiffness and heaviness associated with the increased glycogen storage. Once you start exercising, however, these sensations will work out.

Carbohydrate loading will help only for continuous endurance exercise lasting more than 90 minutes. Greater than usual muscle glycogen stores won't enable you to exercise harder during shorter-duration exercise. In fact, the stiffness and heaviness due to increased glycogen stores can hurt performance during shorter competitions such as 10-kilometer runs.

Carbohydrate loading enables you to maintain high-intensity exercise longer but will not affect your pace for the first hour of exercise. You won't be able to go out faster, but you will be able to maintain your pace longer.

6

PROTEIN:
THE MUSCLE
BUILDER

The Recommended Dietary Allowance (RDA) for protein is 0.8 gram per kilogram per day for sedentary adults. Athletes need more protein—about 50–100% more than the adult RDA. The factors that influence protein requirements include the sport (endurance versus strength), exercise intensity, the carbohydrate content of the diet, level of training, and calorie intake.

This chapter discusses the protein needs of strength and endurance athletes, good food sources of protein, and protein and amino acid supplements.

EXERCISE AND PROTEIN REQUIREMENTS

During endurance exercise, there is an increased breakdown of branched chain amino acids (leucine, isoleucine, and valine) for energy that is proportional to exercise intensity. The hormonal changes that occur with endurance exercise—increased epinephrine (adrenaline) and norepinephrine and decreased insulin—promote increased protein breakdown. Following endurance exercise, however, protein synthesis is increased to minimize and repair any muscle damage that has occurred.

Endurance athletes require about 1.2 to 1.4 grams of protein per kilogram/day.

When muscle glycogen stores are low, due to prolonged exercise or a low-carbohydrate diet, protein may contribute as much as 15% of energy during exercise. When glycogen stores are high, protein utilization decreases to about 5%. Consuming a high-carbohydrate diet during repeated days of heavy training helps maintain glycogen stores and reduces the use of protein as fuel.

During strength exercise such as weight lifting, carbohydrate is your major fuel source. The anaerobic nature of strength exercise minimizes the contribution of amino acids to your fuel needs. However, you do need more protein during strength training to support the higher rates of muscle synthesis induced by this type of exercise. Strength athletes need about 1.6 to 1.7 grams of protein per kilogram/day.

An increased protein intake appears to be more important during the early stages of training than later in the training program. Strength athletes initially need more protein to support increases in their muscle mass—their existing muscle fibers become larger (hypertrophy). Endurance athletes initially need more protein to support increases in the aerobic enzymes (proteins) in the muscle, red blood cell formation, and myoglobin (an oxygen carrier in the muscle similar to hemoglobin).

You may be able to enhance the powerful anabolic stimulus of strength training by consuming carbohydrate immediately after exercise. The increased insulin release in response to the carbohydrate feeding increases the muscles' amino acid uptake and protein synthesis. In addition to promoting glycogen storage, consuming carbohydrate following endurance exercise may help to promote recovery by minimizing and repairing muscle damage.

You can obtain 1.2 to 1.7 grams of protein per kilogram/day when 12–15% of your calories come from protein. However, these guidelines assume that you are consuming sufficient calories (energy). There is an inverse relationship between energy intake and protein need. When you eat enough to fulfill your caloric requirements, you'll generally take in enough protein.

Total calorie intake is more important than protein intake when you're attempting to increase muscle mass. Many athletes mistakenly emphasize protein intake over calorie intake when trying to "bulk up." If you have difficulty gaining weight, you probably aren't eating enough calories.

Some athletes don't eat adequate calories and therefore don't consume enough protein due to heavy training or calorie restriction for low-body-weight sports (wrestling, gymnastics, figure skating, or ballet). Either situation increases the protein requirement because the protein is used for energy rather than for muscle growth and repair. Female athletes are far more likely to consume insufficient calories than male athletes.

You can easily meet your protein requirements through your diet. The average American consumes about 100 grams of protein per day—most from animal sources, which contain all the essential amino acids—for a total protein intake of about 1.4 grams of protein/kilogram.

Athletes consume more protein when their calorie intake increases as a result of training. A 70-kilogram athlete who gradually increases his calorie intake from 2,500 to 3,500 kcal during training would increase his protein intake from 94 to 131 grams/day if 15% of his calories came from protein. His daily protein intake relative to body weight would increase from 1.3 grams to 1.8 grams/kilogram, which would be more than adequate.

Good sources of complete proteins are meat, poultry, fish, dairy products, and eggs. An ounce of meat, poultry, or cheese, or one egg each supply about 7 grams of protein containing all the essential amino acids. Milk and yogurt are also excellent protein sources, with 8 ounces supplying about 8 grams of protein. To reduce dietary fat, choose chicken or turkey without the skin, lean meat, fish, and nonfat or 1% fat dairy products. A list of the protein content of some foods is provided in Table 6-1.

TABLE 6-1
Protein Content in Some Common Foods

Food	Amount	Protein Content (Grams)
Meat, Fish, Poultry		
Lean beef	1 oz	8
Chicken	1 oz	8
Turkey breast	1 oz.	8
Fish	1 oz.	7
Eggs	1	6
Beans, Nuts		
Kidney Beans	½ cup	9
Navy beans	½ cup	7
Garbanzo beans (chick peas)	½ cup	6
Tofu	2 oz.	5
Peanut butter	1 tbsp	4
Dairy		
Low-fat cottage cheese	½ cup	13
Milk, whole, skim	1 cup	8
Yogurt	1 cup	8
Cheddar cheese	1 oz	7
Ice cream	½ cup	4
Frozen yogurt	½ cup	4
American cheese	1 oz.	3
Breads, Cereals, Grains		
Macaroni and cheese	½ cup	9
Spaghetti	1 cup cooked	8
Bagel	2 oz.	6
Raisin Bran	1 oz (⅔ cup)	3
Rice	1 cup cooked	3
Bread	1 slice	2
Vegetables		
Baked potato	1 large	4
Peas, green	½ cup	4
Corn	½ cup	2
Lettuce	¼ head	1
Carrot	1 large	1
Fruits		
Banana, orange	1 medium	1
Apple	1 medium	1

FIGURE 6-1
Food Guide Pyramid for Vegetarian Meal Plannning

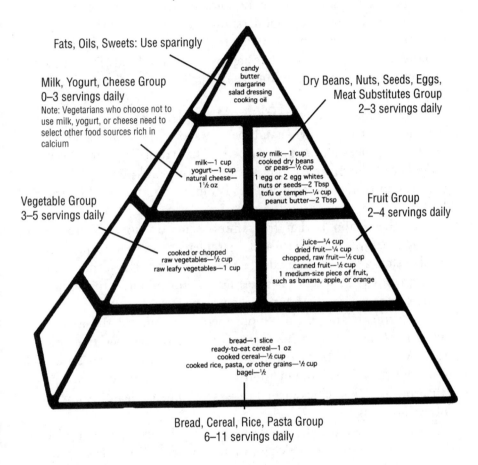

Fats, Oils, Sweets: Use sparingly

candy
butter
margarine
salad dressing
cooking oil

Milk, Yogurt, Cheese Group
0–3 servings daily
Note: Vegetarians who choose not to
use milk, yogurt, or cheese need to
select other food sources rich in
calcium

Dry Beans, Nuts, Seeds, Eggs,
Meat Substitutes Group
2–3 servings daily

milk—1 cup
yogurt—1 cup
natural cheese—
1½ oz

soy milk—1 cup
cooked dry beans
or peas—½ cup
1 egg or 2 egg whites
nuts or seeds—2 Tbsp
tofu or tempeh—¼ cup
peanut butter—2 Tbsp

Vegetable Group
3–5 servings daily

Fruit Group
2–4 servings daily

cooked or chopped
raw vegetables—½ cup
raw leafy vegetables—1 cup

juice—¾ cup
dried fruit—¼ cup
chopped, raw fruit—½ cup
canned fruit—½ cup
1 medium-size piece of fruit,
such as banana, apple, or orange

bread—1 slice
ready-to-eat cereal—1 oz
cooked cereal—½ cup
cooked rice, pasta, or other grains—½ cup
bagel—½

Bread, Cereal, Rice, Pasta Group
6–11 servings daily

Source: National Center for Nutrition and Dietetics
The American Dietetic Association; Based on the USDA Food Guide Pyramid

A well-balanced vegetarian diet can easily supply enough
protein, as long as the protein sources are varied and the athlete
eats enough calories. Guidelines for vegetarians are provided in
Figure 6-1. Whole grains, beans, nuts, seeds, and vegetables supply adequate amounts of essential and nonessential amino acids.

AMINO ACID SUPPLEMENTS

Amino acid supplements containing one or more amino acids are popular among body builders and weight lifters. Proponents of amino acid supplements claim that these products are more rapidly digested and absorbed than protein from food. They may also claim that certain amino acids increase muscle mass and decrease body fat.

The claims made for amino acid supplements are not valid. You may hear that only a small percentage of the amino acids in foods are digested and absorbed. The truth is that about 95–99% of the protein from animal sources and about 90% of the protein from vegetable sources is digested and utilized by the body.

Another claim is that free amino acids do not need to be digested before absorption and so replenish the body's protein pool faster. There is no evidence that more rapid absorption of amino acids is beneficial. It takes hours, not minutes, to rebuild muscle protein damaged during intense exercise.

A further claim is that supplements provide all the amino acids provided by food but are less taxing to the digestive system. Actually, the body readily produces digestive enzymes that systematically break down food protein to amino acids before absorption. Thus, chicken or beans are "timed release" sources of amino acids.

Supplements usually contain 500 milligrams per capsule, while 1 ounce of beef, chicken, or fish supplies 7 grams of protein—7,000 milligrams of amino acids! Compare one cup of a low-fat fruited yogurt that contains 10 grams of high-quality protein, 18 different amino acids (including 300 mg of arginine), carbohydrate, calcium, magnesium, and potassium to one tasteless 500-milligram arginine supplement.

Arginine and ornithine are particularly popular in "fat burner" or "weight gainer" supplements since they supposedly stimulate the secretion of growth hormone—resulting in increased muscle mass and decreased body fat. Although injecting large amounts of arginine and ornithine may cause a temporary rise in growth hormone levels, there is no evidence that the small amounts of these amino acids contained in supplements have any effect on growth hormone levels or body composition. Weight lifting and endurance training both raise growth hormone far more than injecting arginine or ornithine. Combining the supplements with exercise does not increase growth hormone levels above what is seen with exercise.

HIGH-PROTEIN DIETS AND SUPPLEMENTS

Consuming 2 grams of protein per kilogram each day is more than adequate to increase or maintain muscle mass. Going above this amount increases the oxidation (burning) of amino acids. This means that the extra dietary protein will be burned for energy rather than being incorporated into new muscle protein. Using protein for energy is expensive and wasteful. Carbohydrates provide energy more efficiently and at less cost. If you consume enough calories and have a reasonable diet, you'll generally meet or exceed your protein requirements.

Supplemental amino acid or protein intake increases the production of urea, which may increase the risk of becoming dehydrated. The kidneys require more water to eliminate the extra nitrogen load imposed by the excess protein. If you're on a high-protein diet, monitor your body weight daily and drink sufficient fluids to match your losses.

People who have impaired kidney function should not consume large amounts of protein because the added nitrogen excretion increases the kidney's workload. However, there is no good evidence that a high-protein diet is harmful for athletes with healthy kidneys.

There is a concern that high-protein diets may increase calcium loss from the body, thereby increasing the risk of osteoporosis.

Fortunately, the calcium loss observed with purified proteins may be prevented by the increased phosphate intake that occurs with most food proteins.

If your diet provides the recommended amount of protein (1.2 to 1.7 grams per kilogram each day), you probably won't consume an amount of fat that is harmful for your cardiovascular health. To increase your protein intake, choose high-protein foods that are low in saturated fat (nonfat dry milk powder, tuna canned in water, and soy protein powder).

Several best-selling diet books claim that high-protein diets improve athletic performance and promote weight loss. Ketogenic diets (see Chapter 11) are currently popular among many body builders and weight lifters. These diets are very high in saturated fat and may increase the risk of heart disease and stroke. Also, consuming a high-protein, high-fat ketogenic diet after strenuous exercise will cause slow or incomplete replacement of muscle glycogen and impair performance. Ketogenic diets are also hard to digest. By comparison, a high-carbohydrate diet promotes rapid repletion of muscle glycogen and is easy to digest.

Dry milk powder (casein) is a high-quality, inexpensive protein supplement (¼ cup provides 11 grams of protein) that provides all the necessary amino acids at less than half the cost of those heavily advertised "high tech" protein supplements. The "high tech" protein supplements can help you gain weight because they provide additional calories and protein. Although some products contain a variety of ingredients purported to boost weight gain (taurine, whey protein, enzymes), there is no good evidence that these products are superior to protein-rich foods. Nutritional guidelines for gaining weight are discussed in Chapter 11.

Due to the popularity of dietary supplements, it is possible to consume large amounts of single amino acids. This is not possible with protein-rich foods or protein supplements, since both contain a variety of amino acids. With the exception of the eosinophilia-myalgia syndrome (due to contaminated batches of the amino acid tryptophan), there haven't been significant problems with the ingestion of single amino acids. However, large intakes of some single amino acids may interfere with absorption and lead to metabolic imbalances. Ornithine ingestion may cause mild to severe stomach cramping and diarrhea. Other amino acids may alter brain neurotransmitter activity and some, such as methionine, are very toxic. It seems prudent to avoid a large intake of any single amino acid until its safety is determined.

7

FAT:
FRIEND
OR ENEMY?

Most Americans, whether active or sedentary, eat about 34% of their calories as fat. Reducing dietary fat can help to decrease your risk of heart disease (our nation's number one killer), stroke, and certain cancers.

Limiting fat intake is also beneficial for weight control. Fat is the most concentrated source of calories in the diet, supplying twice as many calories by weight as carbohydrate or protein. Dietary fat is also more readily converted to body fat than dietary carbohydrate.

This chapter discusses the importance of fat as a fuel, the health concerns of fat, ways to cut down on fat intake, and how high-fat diets affect performance. Exercise and body fat loss are also addressed.

THE IMPORTANCE OF FAT AS AN EXERCISE FUEL

Whereas the total glycogen stores in your muscle and liver amount to only about 2,000 calories, every pound of fat supplies 3,500 calories. Fat is a major fuel for light- to moderate-intensity exercise.

Even though fat makes significant energy contributions during prolonged endurance exercise, most athletes shouldn't attempt to increase their body fat stores. Most athletes have more body fat stored than they'll ever need, and excess body fat impairs athletic performance. Also, if you eat more fat, you'll eat less carbohydrate. Your muscle glycogen stores cannot be adequately maintained on a high-fat diet.

Remember that endurance training increases your utilization of fat as fuel. The ability to use fat spares muscle glycogen. Since muscle glycogen stores are limited and fat stores are abundant, slowing the rate of glycogen usage improves performance in endurance events such as marathons, bicycle road races, and triathlons.

Proper pacing is also important to maximize fat utilization in endurance events. You'll use less fat and more glycogen by going out too fast and by continuing at a pace that is too fast. Your optimal long-term pace is the speed that allows you to burn more fat and conserve glycogen.

FAT AND HEALTH

Most U.S. health agencies recommend consuming no more than 30% of total calories from fat. Because saturated fat significantly increases the cholesterol level in the blood, it should provide no more than 10% of total calories. Dietary cholesterol should be less than 300 milligrams per day. An elevated blood cholesterol level is a major risk factor for heart disease, as are high blood pressure, inactivity, smoking, and obesity.

The National Cholesterol Education Program defines a desirable blood cholesterol level as below 200 mg/dL (milligrams per deciliter). A blood cholesterol level of 240 mg/dL or more is considered high, and 200 to 239 mg/dL is considered borderline high. These levels are significant, as a cholesterol level of 240 mg/dL doubles the risk of heart disease compared to a cholesterol level of 200 mg/dL.

The way cholesterol is transported in the blood also affects the risk of developing heart disease. Cholesterol is transported in the blood attached to protein as a substance called a lipoprotein. Low-density lipoprotein, or LDL, is the main component of the total cholesterol level. LDL deposits cholesterol in the artery wall and increases the risk of heart disease. High-density lipoprotein, or HDL, on the other hand, removes cholesterol from the artery wall and decreases the risk of heart disease.

An LDL cholesterol level below 130 mg/dL is considered desirable, as shown in Table 7-1. A level of 130 to 159 mg/dL is considered borderline high, and a level of 160 mg/dL is considered high. A high level of HDL cholesterol protects against heart disease, and levels of 60 mg/dL or above significantly decrease heart disease risk. A low level of HDL cholesterol (less than 35 mg/dL) significantly increases the risk of developing heart disease.

In general, decreasing the intake of saturated fat and cholesterol lowers LDL cholesterol and total cholesterol levels. Regular exercise and weight loss raise HDL cholesterol levels.

CUTTING DOWN ON FAT INTAKE

You can obtain a high-carbohydrate, low-fat diet by following the training diet guidelines in Chapter 2. Here are further recommendations to cut down on fat intake:

You can lower your fat intake by cutting down on both "hidden" and "visible" sources of fat. Fat is hidden in dairy products, meat, eggs, nuts, and fried foods. Be aware of the hidden fat in favorite foods such as ice cream, cheese, french fries, chips, granola, cold cuts, bacon, nuts, hamburger, and baked goods (cookies, pies, cakes, and pastries). Visible dietary sources of fat include margarine, butter, cream, mayonnaise, oil, salad dressing, gravies, sauces, sour cream, and cream cheese.

You can reduce your intake of total fat, saturated fat, and cholesterol by choosing lean meat, poultry, and fish. Try to eat

---

TABLE 7-1
It Pays to Know Your Blood Cholesterol Level

BLOOD CHOLESTEROL LEVEL (MG/DL)

< (less than) 200 . . . . .Desirable level
200–239 . . . . .Borderline-high level
> (more than) 239 . . . . .High level

RECOMMENDED FOLLOW-UP

Total cholesterol < 200 mg/dL . . . . . .Repeat within 5 years

Total cholesterol 200–239 mg/dL
Without existent heart disease . . . . . . .Blood cholesterol rechecked annually
or 2 heart-disease risk factors

With 2 other heart-disease . . . . .Lipoprotein analysis: further action
risk factors .based on LDL cholesterol level

Total cholesterol > 239 mg/dL, ...Same as for previous group
regardless of other factors

LDL CHOLESTEROL LEVELS (MG/DL)

< 130 . . . . .Desirable level
130–159 . . . . .Borderline-high level
≥159 . . . . .High-risk level

RISK FACTORS FOR HEART DISEASE

Positive Risk Factors
   Age
   • Male ≥ 45 years
   • Female ≥ 55 years or early menopause without estrogen-replacement therapy
   • Family history of premature heart disease (definite myocardial infarction
     or sudden death before 55 years of age in father or before 65 years of age
     in mother)
   • Current cigarette smoking
   • Hypertension (≥ 140/90 mm Hg or on blood pressure medication)
   • Low HDL cholesterol (< 35 mg/dL)
   • Diabetes

Negative Risk Factors
   High HDL cholesterol (≥ 60 mg/dL)

---

less high-fat processed meat such as bologna, bacon, salami, and hot dogs. Removing the skin from poultry and trimming visible fat from meat also cuts down on fat. The Dietary Guidelines recommend consuming 5 to 7 ounces of meat, poultry, or fish per day.

The butterfat found in butter, cheese, chocolate, ice cream, and whole milk can also be limited to reduce your intake of total fat, saturated fat, and cholesterol. Substitute nonfat and low-fat dairy products such as 1% fat milk and yogurt, ice milk, and low-fat cheese for high-fat dairy products. The Dietary Guidelines recommend consuming two to three servings of dairy products each day.

Oils with high percentages of unsaturated fat (canola, corn, olive, and soy oil and their derivative margarines) should be substituted for saturated fats such as butter, lard, shortening, and bacon grease. When oil and margarine are substituted for butter, remember that they are still high in fat and calories and should be used sparingly. Reduced-fat substitutes for salad dressing and sour cream can replace the higher-fat versions.

Choose cooking methods that require little or no fat. These include steaming, baking, broiling, grilling, poaching, or stir-frying in small amounts of unsaturated vegetable oil. Foods can be microwaved or cooked in pans that have been sprayed with non-stick products to reduce added fat. Try to limit fried foods, especially when saturated fat is used.

Although nonfat and low-fat bakery goods and frozen dairy products contain little or no fat, they do contain calories. Remember to check the food label—fat-free does not mean calorie-free. These products can be loaded with extra sugar (calories) and sodium to improve taste.

HIGH-FAT DIETS AND PERFORMANCE

High-fat diets are sometimes promoted to improve performance. The claim is that "fat loading" enables you to burn fat, rather than glycogen, as your major fuel source. Because fat

TABLE 7-2
How to Reduce Dietary Fat and Cholesterol

	CHOOSE	DECREASE
Fish, Chicken, Turkey, and Lean Meats	Fish, poultry without skin, lean cuts of beef, lamb, pork, or veal, shellfish	Fatty cuts of beef, lamb, pork; spare ribs, organ meats regular cold cuts, sausage, hot dogs, bacon, sardines, roe
Skim and Low-fat Milk, Cheese, Yogurt, and Dairy Substitutes	Skim or 1% fat milk (liquid, powdered, evaporated), buttermilk	Whole milk (4% fat); regular, evaporated, condensed; cream, half and half, 2% milk, imitation milk products, most nondairy creamers, whipped toppings
	Nonfat (0% fat) or low-fat yogurt Nonfat or low-fat cottage cheese (1% or 2% fat)	Whole-milk yogurt Whole-milk cottage cheese (4% fat)
	Nonfat, low-fat cheeses (0–6 gm fat/ounce)	All natural cheeses (e.g., blue, roquefort, camembert, cheddar, swiss)
	Nonfat, low-fat, or "light" cream cheese, nonfat, low-fat, or "light" sour cream	Cream cheeses, sour cream
	Nonfat, low-fat ice cream Sherbet Sorbet Nonfat, low-fat frozen yogurt	Regular ice cream
Eggs	Egg whites (2 whites = 1 whole egg in recipes), cholesterol-free egg substitutes	Egg yolks

---

TABLE 7-2 (continued)
How to Reduce Dietary Fat and Cholesterol

	CHOOSE	DECREASE
Fruits and Vegetables	Fresh, frozen, canned, or dried fruits and vegetables	Vegetables prepared in butter, cheese, cream, or other creamy sauces
Breads and Cereals	Homemade baked goods using unsaturated oils sparingly, angel food cake, nonfat or low-fat crackers, nonfat or low-fat cookies	Commercial baked goods: pies, cakes, donuts, pastries, croissants, muffins, biscuits, high-fat crackers, high-fat cookies
	Rice, pasta	Egg noodles
	Whole-grain breads and cereals (oatmeal, whole wheat, rye, bran, multigrain, etc.)	Breads in which eggs are major ingredient
Fats and Oils	Baking cocoa	Chocolate
	Unsaturated vegetable oils; corn, olive, rapeseed (canola oil), safflower, sesame, soybean, sunflower	Saturated oils: butter, coconut, palm, palm kernel, lard, bacon fat
	Liquid, tub margarine or shortening made from one of the unsaturated oils listed above	Stick margarine
	Diet margarine	
	Low-fat or nonfat mayonnaise, salad dressings made with unsaturated oils listed above	Dressings made with egg yolk
	Nonfat or low-fat dressings	Regular dressings
	Seeds and nuts	Coconut

stores are plentiful and glycogen stores are limited, fat loading supposedly enhances performance.

There is no convincing evidence that a high-fat diet improves performance. In fact, just the opposite is likely to occur. Eating too much fat decreases intake of carbohydrate and reduces glycogen stores. Carbohydrate, not fat, is the preferred fuel during the high-exercise intensities at which most athletes train and compete. The bottom line: A high-fat diet will impair performance.

The other drawbacks of high-fat diets outweigh any potential benefits. Such diets need medical supervision—they have been associated with sudden death and heart rhythm disturbances due to protein and potassium losses.

The blood cholesterol level can rise on a high-fat diet despite heavy training. Because exercise by itself doesn't prevent heart disease, eating a high-fat diet for a long time may increase the risk of developing heart disease.

A high-fat diet takes longer to digest, which is one of the reasons fat should be limited in the pre-exercise meal. Examples of "fat loading" meals include cheese, marbled or ground beef, eggs, butter, and tuna mixed with mayonnaise. Such a diet isn't palatable and lacks the variety of nutrients you need for optimal performance.

Adapting to a high-fat diet takes at least two weeks. During this time, exercising will be difficult and unpleasant due to low muscle glycogen stores. Even after adaptation is complete, you won't be able to sustain the high intensity required for most competitions.

It makes no sense to adjust to a high-fat diet when you can get immediate performance benefits from a high-carbohydrate diet. Your ability to burn fat is increased far more effectively by endurance training than by eating a high-fat diet.

EXERCISE AND BODY FAT LOSS

Some believe that individuals who want to lose body fat should exercise at a lower intensity since fat contributes more to the metabolic mixture. Unfortunately, this assumption misses the whole point: Regular exercise is beneficial for weight loss because it creates a prolonged calorie deficit.

The fuel being burned to create this calorie deficit (fat or carbohydrate) is not important. There is no scientific evidence that using fat as fuel will produce greater body fat loss than using carbohydrate as fuel. It is the calorie deficit that is important.

Although a greater percentage of fat may be burned with low-intensity exercise, the total amount of fat burned is actually greater with high-intensity exercise because the total energy expenditure is higher during intense activity. The fuel burned during exercise (carbohydrate or fat) doesn't matter when the goal is to lose weight.

In other words, low-intensity exercise uses a greater percentage of fat than high-intensity exercise, but the fat calories (and carbohydrate calories) are being burned at a relatively slow rate —4 to 5 calories per minute.

By comparison, high-intensity exercise uses a smaller percentage of fat, but this smaller percentage (along with carbohydrate) is burned at a much higher rate—10 to 15 calories per minute. So, the total amount of fat burned is greater at the higher-intensity levels.

Many individuals have confused the proportion of fat used as fuel with the more important rate of fuel utilization, which is a key concept in exercise-induced body fat loss. When the goal of an exercise program is to lose weight, the exercise should create a calorie deficit. To lose 1 pound of body fat, an individual must expend 3,500 calories, whether those calories come from fat or carbohydrate.

The person's fitness level must be considered when exercise is recommended as part of a weight-loss program. Low- to moderate-intensity exercise is recommended for overweight people who are just starting to exercise. High-intensity exercise is associated with an increased risk of orthopedic injuries. Also, unfit people who engage in high-intensity exercise usually find it unpleasant and may stop exercising altogether.

Individuals who are just starting to exercise for weight loss should exercise at a lower intensity. The only drawback of low-intensity exercise is that the person must exercise longer to achieve a significant calorie deficit. Other than that, a low-intensity workout that expends 300 calories in 1 hour is just as beneficial for body fat loss as a high-intensity workout that expends 300 calories in 30 minutes.

8

VITAMINS AND MINERALS: HELP OR HYPE?

M any active people take vitamin and mineral supplements for "nutritional insurance" to compensate for less-than-adequate diets or lifestyles, to meet the unusual demands imposed by heavy exercise, or to improve their performance.

This chapter discusses the Dietary Reference Intakes for vitamins and minerals, supplementation concerns, supplement recommendations, and the antioxidant vitamins C and E. Iron and calcium are minerals of specific concern for athletes and are also addressed.

DIETARY REFERENCE INTAKES

The Dietary Reference Intakes (DRIs) are nutrient-based reference values that expand and replace the Recommended Dietary Allowances (RDAs) published since 1941 by the Food and Nutrition Board of the National Academy of Sciences. The DRIs represent a shift in emphasis from preventing nutritional deficiency to decreasing the risk of chronic disease. When adequate scientific evidence exists, the DRIs include levels that may help to prevent diet-related diseases such as cardiovascular disease, certain cancers, and osteoporosis.

The DRIs include RDAs as goals for daily intake by individuals but present three new categories of reference values:

Estimated average requirement (EAR)—the intake that meets the estimated nutrient need of 50% of the individuals in a specific age and gender group. This figure is used to help develop the RDA and may also be used to evaluate the adequacy of nutrient intakes for population groups.

Recommended Dietary Allowance (RDA)—the intake that meets the estimated nutrient need of nearly all (97–98%) healthy individuals in a specific age and gender group. The RDA value will help guide individuals to achieve adequate nutrient intake.

Adequate Intake (AI)—used when sufficient scientific evidence is not available to calculate an estimated average requirement. The AI value is used as a goal for individual dietary intake when an RDA cannot be determined. The DRI committee set AIs for calcium, vitamin D, and fluoride.

Tolerable Upper Intake Level (UL)—the maximum intake that is unlikely to pose risks of adverse health effects in nearly all individuals in a specified group. As intake increases above the UL, the risk of adverse effects increases. The UL is not intended to be a recommended level of intake. The DRI committee set ULs for many nutrients, including vitamin D, niacin, and vitamin B_6. For some nutrients, there may be insufficient data to develop a UL. This doesn't mean that the nutrient isn't potentially harmful at high levels of intake.

VITAMIN/MINERAL NEEDS OF ATHLETES

In small amounts, vitamins function as catalysts—substances that increase the speed of a reaction without being used up by the reaction. The fact that vitamins aren't used up explains why they are needed only in small amounts.

Contrary to popular belief, vitamins do not provide energy, although the B vitamins are important for the release of energy

FIGURE 8-1
The B Vitamins

The B vitamins are important for the release of energy
from carbohydrate in the muscle cell.

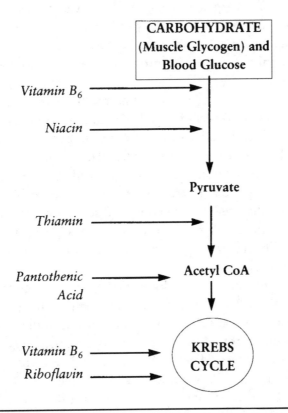

from carbohydrates, fats, and proteins (see Figure 8-1). Only carbohydrate, fat, and protein provide energy (calories). This means that in general the vitamin requirements of an active person are not significantly higher than those of a sedentary person.

The B vitamins thiamin, riboflavin, and niacin are required in proportion to calories consumed, and active people need more calories. However, a balanced diet provides ample amounts of these vitamins. They are supplied by those carbohydrate-rich foods recommended for athletes—bread and whole-grain or enriched-grain products.

You may feel that taking vitamin/mineral supplements is justified because the DRIs don't account for the varying nutritional needs of different people. In general, the nutrient needs for the average person are only about two-thirds of the RDA or AI. This means that as long as you consume at least 67% of the RDA or AI for a given nutrient, you are probably protected from a nutritional deficiency.

Supplementation at levels exceeding the RDA or AI does not improve the performance of well-nourished athletes. Although vitamin and mineral deficiencies can impair performance, it is very unusual for athletes to have such deficiencies. There is a close relationship between calorie intake and vitamin intake—the more food eaten, the greater the vitamin intake. Athletes generally eat more than sedentary people and so tend to obtain more vitamins and minerals in relation to their needs. Also, the carbohydrate-rich diet recommended for athletes contains foods with high nutrient density.

Athletes who limit their calorie intake are at risk for nutritional deficiencies. These athletes usually compete in sports that emphasize leanness for enhanced performance (distance runners, wrestlers, lightweight crew) or for appearance (gymnasts, dancers, figure skaters, divers). Weight-conscious active people may also be at risk. A vitamin/mineral supplement supplying 100% of the RDA or AI may be appropriate for these individuals.

Athletes often feel that "staleness" or "flatness" is due to a vitamin or mineral deficiency. When there is a nutritional reason for fatigue, it is usually an inadequate intake of calories or carbohydrate. If you're always tired, you may be overtraining or eating too little carbohydrate or calories for glycogen synthesis. If you feel better after taking vitamin/mineral supplements, it's probably due to the strength of your belief that the supplements helped—the "placebo effect."

IRON

Iron is an essential trace element required for the formation of hemoglobin and myoglobin—the oxygen-carrying components of red blood cells and muscle cells. Two-thirds of the total amount of iron in the body is in hemoglobin. When the total hemoglobin concentration drops, the muscles do not receive as much oxygen.

Iron deserves particular attention in the athlete's diet due to the prevalence of iron-deficiency anemia—the nation's most common nutritional deficiency. Women are much more likely to suffer from iron-deficiency anemia due to menstrual blood losses and inadequate iron intake.

Iron deficiency occurs in three stages. Low levels of hemoglobin (below 12 gm/dL for women and 13 gm/dL for men) are diagnostic indicators for iron-deficiency anemia, the third stage of iron deficiency. Since most of the oxygen transported in the blood is bound to the iron in hemoglobin, it is not surprising that iron-deficiency anemia reduces both maximum aerobic capacity and endurance. Table 8-1 shows the progression of iron deficiency to anemia.

Exercise may increase iron excretion and so increase the risk of developing iron deficiency in both men and women. Excessive iron losses during exercise are most likely to occur through gastrointestinal bleeding and sweating. Some female athletes (distance runners) also consume foods with low iron bioavailability and are at increased risk of depleting their iron stores.

Female and male athletes must take special care to consume the RDA for iron—18 mg for women and 10 mg for men. Iron intake averages 6 mg of iron per 1,000 kcal. Whereas male athletes usually consume more iron than the RDA, female athletes tend to consume less iron than the RDA. This is especially true in the aesthetic sports (gymnastics, ballet) where the female athlete restricts calories to maintain a lower body weight.

Athletes at risk for iron deficiency, particularly menstruating women, should have routine checks of their iron status. Plasma

TABLE 8-1
Progression of Iron Deficiency to Anemia

Progression	Method of Detection	Hematologic Profile
Iron depletion	Serum ferritin	Depletion of iron stores in liver, bone marrow, and spleen
Iron-deficiency erythropoiesis	Serum iron, total iron-binding capacity, transferrin saturation	Depleted iron stores, decreased levels of plasma iron, increased hepatic formation of transferrin
		Increase of total iron-binding capacity to 400–500 mcg/dL
		Fall of percent transferrin saturation from mean of 30% to about 15–18%
Iron-deficiency anemia	HGB, RBC count hematocrit, mean cell hemoglobin concentration	Fall of hemoglobin concentration to below 12 gm/dL

Source: Adapted from Physician Sportsmed., 1984.

ferritin (storage iron) and transferrin (transport iron) saturation should be measured in addition to hemoglobin. Although more expensive, these tests are valuable because they can detect iron deficiency early. A low plasma ferritin level and decreased transferrin saturation mean that the athlete is at greater risk of developing iron-deficiency anemia. The athlete's iron stores can be increased through diet and/or iron supplementation to prevent the negative consequences of iron-deficiency anemia.

While iron-deficiency anemia impairs performance, iron depletion without anemia does not. Iron supplements won't improve the health or performance of an athlete with normal hemoglobin levels. If iron supplements are used, they shouldn't exceed the RDA unless medically indicated and prescribed by a physician.

Obtaining Adequate Iron

The iron from animal iron sources (heme iron) is absorbed better than the iron from vegetable iron sources (non-heme iron). Red meat is an excellent iron source, containing about 1 milligram of iron per ounce. Combining animal and vegetable products (meat and bean burrito) increases the iron absorbed from the vegetable product. Vitamin C also enhances non-heme iron absorption, so high vitamin C foods (orange juice) should be consumed with foods containing non-heme iron (iron fortified cereals) for optimum absorption.

Iron-enriched or fortified cereal/grain products can contribute significantly to the iron content of the diet. Beans, peas, split peas, and some dark-green leafy vegetables are good vegetable iron sources. Cast iron cookware also increases the iron content of foods. The more acidic and the longer the food is cooked in cast iron (e.g., spaghetti sauce), the higher the residual iron content of the food. Table 8-2 lists good sources of iron and the milligrams of iron each provides.

CALCIUM

Calcium, the most abundant mineral in the body, is critical for the conduction of nerve impulses, heart function, muscle contraction, and the operation of certain enzymes. The bones and teeth contain 99% of the body's calcium; the remaining 1% circulates in the bloodstream. When the supply of calcium in the blood is too low, the body withdraws calcium from the bones.

TABLE 8-2
Food Sources for Iron

Each serving size listed contains at least 1.5 milligrams of iron

Food	Serving Size	Food	Serving Size
Apricots, dried	5 halves	Peaches, dried	2 halves
Beans, dried	½ cup	Peanut butter	5 tbs.
Beet greens, cooked	½ cup	Peas	⅔ cup
Cereals#, bran 40%	1 oz.	Peas, dried	⅛ cup
Chickpeas or garbanzos	⅛ cup	Poultry:	
Cider, sweet	10 oz.	Chicken, cooked	3½ oz.
Egg, whole (medium)	2	Turkey, cooked	3½ oz.
Fig bars	4 large	Prunes, dried	4 medium
Fish:		Prune juice	¼ cup
Sardines (canned)*	2 oz.	Raisins, dried	1½ oz.
Scallops	2 oz.	Soybeans	2 oz.
Shrimp	2 oz.	Soybean curd (tofu)	¼ cup
Tuna (canned)*	½ cup	Spinach, raw, frozen	2 oz.
Grits	¼ cup	Spinach, cooked, canned#	½ cup
Instant Breakfast*+	1 serving	Strawberries	1 cup
Lentils, cooked	3 oz.	Tomato juice (canned)*	¾ cup
Maple syrup	3 tbs.	Watermelon	6" diameter
Meat:			x 1½" slice
Beef, chipped or dried*+	1 oz.	Wheat germ	2 tbs.
Beef, cooked+	2 oz.		
Ham, cooked, cured*+	2 oz.		
Lamb, cooked+	3 oz.		
Molasses	2 Tbs.		
Mustard greens	⅔ cup		
Nuts:			
Brazil nuts	½ cup		
Peanuts, roasted*	⅔ cup	* = High in sodium	
Pecans	⅔ cup	+ = High in cholesterol or saturated fat	
Pinenuts, piñon nuts	¾ oz.	# = Not well metabolized	
Pistachio nuts	¼ oz.		
Walnuts	½ cup of halves		

An adequate intake of calcium is an important nutritional strategy in the prevention of osteoporosis, an age-related disorder in which bone mass decreases and the susceptibility to fractures increases. Osteoporosis is called the "silent disease" because it usually progresses painlessly until a fracture occurs, typically in the hip, wrist, or spine.

Osteoporosis cannot be cured—it can only be prevented or its progression delayed. A well-balanced, calcium-rich diet and regular exercise help to decrease the risk of osteoporosis. Dual x-ray absorptiometry is an accurate way to measure bone mineral mass and so detect osteoporosis early, with minimal radiation exposure.

Women are more susceptible to osteoporosis because of their lower bone mineral density and total bone mass. Also, after menopause women produce less estrogen, which further accelerates bone loss.

Dietary calcium exerts its greatest effect on bone mineral density from preadolescence to young adulthood. Until peak bone mass is attained at approximately 30 years of age, bone formation exceeds the rate of bone resorption. The amount of bone mass an individual has by age 30 will strongly influence susceptibility to fractures in later years.

All athletes should consume the recommended amount of calcium to promote optimal bone health. The Adequate Intake, or AI, values for calcium are 800 milligrams per day for children ages 4 to 8, 1,300 milligrams for children and adolescents ages 9 to 18, 1,000 milligrams for adults 19 to 50, and 1,200 milligrams for adults over 50. Women, in particular, fall short. Female adolescents who have a poor calcium intake and amenorrheic athletes are a special concern because they may be setting themselves up for an increased risk of subsequent osteoporosis.

Obtaining Adequate Calcium

Dairy products are the best sources of calcium. An 8-ounce glass of milk or ⅓ cup of nonfat powdered milk each contains about 300 milligrams of calcium. Skim or low-fat versions of milk, yogurt, cottage cheese, or cheese often provide the same amount of calcium as the regular versions of these foods, but contain less fat and calories.

Other good sources of calcium are sardines (because of the bones) and oysters. Broccoli and greens (kale, collard, turnip, and mustard) are good sources of calcium without any fat. Tofu that has been processed with calcium sulfate can also be a good source of calcium. Table 8-3 lists good sources of calcium and the milligrams of calcium each provides.

Many other nutrients influence calcium absorption and bone formation. Vitamin D is important for bone health because its active form stimulates the absorption of calcium from the intestine. However, high intakes of protein, sodium, and caffeine interfere with calcium retention by increasing the amount of calcium excreted in the urine. Excessive alcohol intake also has detrimental effects on bone mass.

A registered dietitian can provide advice on how to obtain the appropriate amount of calcium from food and supplements. Calcium carbonate (Tums or a generic equivalent) is an inexpensive and acceptable calcium source. Calcium carbonate is 40% calcium, so a 500-mg tablet actually provides 200 milligrams of elemental calcium. Such antacids that contain calcium are practically the same as dietary supplements. The primary difference between the two is in the marketing—when calcium carbonate is marketed as a calcium supplement, it costs more.

Too much calcium can be harmful. In susceptible people, excessive calcium intake increases the risk of kidney stones. Excessive calcium from diet or supplements may also interfere with the absorption of iron. The adult Upper Limit, or UL, for calcium is 2.5 grams per day.

SUPPLEMENTATION CONCERNS

High doses of vitamins and minerals (amounts above the Tolerable Upper Intake Level) can be dangerous. Consuming large amounts of vitamins and minerals can produce serious side effects and upset the delicate balance of these nutrients.

TABLE 8-3
Food Sources for Calcium

Food	Serving Size	Micrograms of Calcium
Milk and dairy products:		
Milk, LactAid Calcium		
Fortified Nonfat	1 cup	500
Yogurt, nonfat, plain	1 cup	452
yogurt, low-fat, plain	1 cup	415
Milk, skim, protein-fortified	1 cup	352
Milk, skim, regular	1 cup	302
*Swiss cheese	1 oz.	272
*Mozzarella, part skim	1 oz.	207
*Cheddar cheese	1 oz.	204
*Ricotta cheese, part skim	1 oz.	169
Ice cream or ice milk	1 cup	164
*Cottage cheese, 2% low-fat	1 cup	154
Tofu	3 oz.	150
*Parmesan cheese, grated	1 tbsp.	69
Bread and Grain Products:		
Wonder Calcium-Enriched Bread	2 slices	580
Total cereal	¾ cup	250
Bread, white or whole wheat	2 slices	47
Fruits and Juices		
Tropicana Season's Best Orange	1 cup	333
Juice Plus Calcium		
Minute Maid Calcium-Enriched	1 cup	293
Orange Juice		
Orange	1 medium	52
Fish:		
*Sardines, canned in water, drained	2 oz.	185
*Salmon, canned, drained	3 oz.	167
Vegetables		
Collards, frozen	½ cup, cooked	179
Turnip greens, chopped	½ cup, cooked	99
Kale, frozen	½ cup, cooked	90

(continued on next page)

TABLE 8-3 (continued)
Food Sources for Calcium

Food	Serving Size	Micrograms of Calcium
Vegetables (continued)		
Bok choy	½ cup, cooked	79
Swiss chard, chopped	½ cup, cooked	49
Broccoli, chopped	½ cup, cooked	36
Sweet potato, baked	1 medium	32
Nuts and Legumes:		
Almonds	½ cup	150
Soybeans	½ cup, cooked	88
Pinto beans	½ cup, cooked	41

* = High in sodium

Sources:
USDA *Handbook 8* and Bowes and Church, *Food Values of Portions Commonly Used.*

As mentioned in Chapter 1, fat-soluble vitamins (A and D in particular) can build up in the body to toxic levels. Large doses of water-soluble vitamins can also cause side effects. Some body builders take large doses of niacin (a B vitamin) to make their blood vessels dilate and stand out. However, large amounts of niacin can cause severe flushing, skin disorders, liver damage, ulcers, and blood sugar disorders. High doses of niacin also interfere with fat metabolism and speed up glycogen depletion.

Niacin may be useful in the treatment of elevated blood cholesterol and triglycerides. However, it should never be used for this purpose without medical supervision. Large doses of vitamin C have been associated with diarrhea, kidney stone formation, and impaired copper absorption.

Vitamin B_6 (pyridoxine) toxicity has been documented in women who have taken supplements to alleviate premenstrual symptoms. Excess vitamin B_6 can cause neurological symptoms similar to multiple sclerosis, including numbness and tingling of the hands, difficulty in walking, and electric shocks shooting down the spine. Toxicity has been reported in people taking as little as 200 milligrams—the RDA for vitamin B_6 is about 1.3 milligrams.

Like fat-soluble vitamins, excess amounts of minerals are stored in the body and can gradually build up to toxic levels. An excess of one mineral can also interfere with the functioning of others. A high iron intake, for example, can produce an iron overload (hemochromatosis) in genetically predisposed people and cause deficiencies of other trace minerals (zinc and copper). If untreated, iron overload can damage the liver, pancreas, and heart. Although iron deficiency affects far more people than iron overload, iron supplements should be used only for proven iron deficiency.

SUPPLEMENT RECOMMENDATIONS

There is no established benefit for individuals to consume nutrients at levels above the RDA or AI. The Committee on Diet and Health (Food and Nutrition Board, National Research Council) recommends that people avoid taking dietary supplements that exceed 100% of the RDA or AI in any one day. Most people can, and should, obtain essential nutrients from a variety of foods.

The Committee noted possible exceptions in the cases of women who are pregnant or breast-feeding, women with excess monthly bleeding, people on very-low-calorie diets, some vegetarians, and people with malabsorption problems. However, rather than automatically taking vitamin/mineral supplements, these individuals should be evaluated on a case-by-case basis.

For active people and athletes who do not fit into any of these categories, most health authorities agree that there is no harm in taking a simple vitamin/mineral supplement, provided that it does not exceed 100% of the RDA or AI for nutrients. There is, however, no evidence to prove that such supplementation is beneficial.

To ensure a high-quality vitamin/mineral supplement, look for products that have USP (United States Pharmacopeia) on the supplement label. This means that the supplement company is legally responsible to the Food and Drug Administration for meeting USP dissolution standards—the standard for how well a supplement dissolves. The USP also means that the supplement has gone through a battery of other tests as well—disintegration, strength (potency), and purity. It also helps to look for nationally known food and drug manufacturers who make their products under the tight manufacturing controls that they already have in place.

It's much easier to take a vitamin/mineral supplement than to improve food selection and eating habits. However, you can't improve your performance simply by taking a pill. Just as an adequate diet isn't improved by supplements, an inadequate diet isn't "fixed" by supplements.

Consuming a variety of foods from the Food Guide Pyramid each day reduces the need for vitamin/mineral supplementation. Whereas different foods contain a variety of nutrients and other compounds (dietary fiber, phytochemicals) that promote health, supplements don't usually contain these compounds. If you want "nutritional insurance," eat more nutrient-dense grain products, fruits, vegetables, and legumes and fewer empty calories such as sugar, fat, and alcohol.

ANTIOXIDANTS

Many people take antioxidant supplements such as vitamins C and E to protect against heart disease, cancer, and other chronic diseases associated with aging. Some active people and athletes also use antioxidants to reduce the amount of muscle damage and soreness caused by heavy exercise.

Free radicals, substances that can cause damage to muscle cells and cell membranes, are released by the body's own normal process of producing energy. Exercise causes a number of physiological changes that increase the production of free radicals. These include an elevated metabolic rate, increased body temperature, and higher epinephrine levels. The production of free radicals can also be increased by exposure to various environmental pollutants such as smog, cigarette smoke, radiation, and certain pesticides.

Fortunately, the body possesses its own antioxidant defense of enzymes (catalase, superoxide dismutase, and glutathione peroxidase) and obtains the antioxidant vitamins E and C through diet. Each of these antioxidants works at different sites within the body and in a different manner from each other. Their overall goal, however, is to stop the production and spread of harmful free-radical chain reactions.

Vitamin E helps to protect structures that contain lipids (such as cell membranes) from free-radical attack. Vitamin C works to stop free radicals within the water compartments found within and between the cells. In addition to being an antioxidant nutrient by itself, vitamin C can regenerate vitamin E.

Regular physical training itself provides a partially protective effect. Consistent workouts increase the activity of the enzymes that clean up the free radicals, thereby helping to minimize muscle damage.

While antioxidant supplements may protect against muscle damage, they won't help the performance of adequately nourished athletes. For example, vitamin E deficiency does impair endurance capacity, and this is associated with greater free-radical damage. However, vitamin E supplementation doesn't improve aerobic capacity or endurance in well-nourished athletes.

Vitamin E supplementation may reduce free-radical production and lessen muscle damage following heavy, unaccustomed exercise such as downhill running or skiing. Vitamin C may alleviate muscle soreness and enhance the return of muscle function following such hard, unusual exercise.

Your age may also determine whether antioxidant supplements are beneficial. Vitamin E was found to stimulate the rate of muscle repair after exercise-induced muscle damage in older, but not younger, individuals.

The RDAs for vitamin C (75 milligrams for adult women and 90 milligrams for adult men) and vitamin E (15 milligrams, or 22 International Units) can be readily obtained through a varied diet that emphasizes plant foods.

Populations who eat adequate amounts of fruits and vegetables have a lower incidence of heart disease, certain cancers, and cataracts. While fruits and vegetables are rich in antioxidants, they also provide other nutrients, fiber, and phytochemicals that are beneficial for health. Regardless of supplements, all active people will benefit from consuming the recommended amount of vegetables (three to four servings) and fruit (two to four servings) a day.

Athletes should avoid taking large doses of the minerals that work with the free-radical-suppressing enzymes—zinc, copper, and selenium. Excess zinc consumption may reduce HDL cholesterol levels, impair immune function, and inhibit copper absorption from foods, possibly leading to anemia. Copper supplements aren't recommended since athletes don't appear to be deficient and there's no evidence to suggest that copper will enhance performance.

Selenium is a particular supplement favorite, since it works with vitamin E to protect cell membranes against free-radical damage. However, research suggests that vitamin E, rather than selenium, is crucial for protection against free-radical damage. There is no reason to take selenium supplements as most people get enough selenium and an excess intake may be harmful.

9

FLUID REQUIREMENTS AND HYDRATION

Water is the most essential of all nutrients since your body requires it constantly. All the body's important chemical reactions, such as energy production, are carried out in water. Without water, most people could not survive for more than a few days.

Although water has a number of important functions, the most critical function for athletes is the regulation of body temperature. Consuming cool fluids at regular intervals during exercise protects your health and optimizes athletic performance.

This chapter discusses the distribution of water in the body, the importance of water for temperature regulation during exercise, heat illnesses, and fluid-replacement guidelines, fluid-replacement beverages, and electrolytes (sodium and potassium). The chapter also reviews the effects of alcoholic and caffeinated beverages on performance.

DISTRIBUTION OF BODY WATER

Water is stored in several areas of the body but moves continually between these areas. About 65% of the body's water is stored inside the cells as intracellular water. The remaining 35%

is stored outside the cells as extracellular water. The extracellular water is divided into the interstitial water between or surrounding the cells and the vascular water within the circulating blood.

Proper water and electrolyte balance within these areas is extremely important. Fluid shifts such as decreases in the blood volume and cellular dehydration can occur from sweat losses during exercise in hot, dry weather. This contributes to fatigue and increases the risk of developing heat illnesses.

Water makes up about 60% of the body weight in the average adult male and about 50% in the adult female. This percentage may be as low as 40% in obese individuals and as high as 70% in muscular ones. This is because fat tissue is low in water (about 10–15%) and muscle tissue is high in water (about 70–75%). Thus, athletes who have a high muscle mass and low fat content have a relatively high body-water content.

WATER AND TEMPERATURE
REGULATION DURING EXERCISE

Water acts as a coolant to keep the body from overheating during physical activity. During exercise, heat is generated as a by-product of the working muscles. When heat builds up, the body temperature rises. This heat must be removed to maintain a normal body temperature.

During exercise in warm weather, sweat is your main way to eliminate excess heat. When sweat evaporates from the skin, you cool down. Large sweat losses, however, reduce your body's water content. The loss of water in sweat harms your athletic performance and hinders your ability to control body temperature.

During exercise on hot days, blood that was transferring oxygen to the muscles is diverted to skin to help eliminate heat. The competition for blood between the muscles and skin places a greater demand on the cardiovascular system. At the same time, blood volume is decreasing due to sweat losses. As the body becomes dehydrated, heart rate, perceived level of effort, and body temperature all increase.

The fluid in sweat initially comes from the extracellular fluid compartments: blood plasma and interstitial fluid. Eventually, intracellular fluid will also be reduced as the increase in extracellular sodium levels draws water from the intracellular space. The muscle and skin contribute about 70% of the total water lost in sweat, which may protect the brain and other vital organs.

Your body is programmed to protect cardiovascular function at the expense of body temperature regulation. Consequently, skin blood flow and sweat rate are decreased in an effort to conserve body fluid. As a result, body temperature rises, leading to fatigue and increased risk of heat injury.

In practical terms, when you're dehydrated you can't exercise as hard or as long. Sweat losses constituting as little as 2% of body weight impair athletic performance and temperature regulation during prolonged exercise in the heat. Inadequate fluid replacement speeds up dehydration and can ultimately cause a life-threatening heat illness.

WEATHER CONCERNS

You may be unaware of the enormous sweat losses that can occur during hot, dry weather. Large amounts of fluid evaporate very quickly in these conditions. Since you don't feel sweaty, you may not recognize how much water you've lost.

Besides heat, relative humidity is also important. As the moisture in the air increases, the effectiveness of heat loss through sweating decreases. If the air is saturated with water, little evaporation will occur even at cooler temperatures and body heat can build up. When the sweat drips off your skin, you're not getting the cooling benefit of evaporation. Be aware of intense physical exertion on warm, humid days, as well as on hot, dry days (see Table 9-1).

TABLE 9-1
Heat Index

TEMPERATURE

Relative Humidity	70°	75°	80°	85°	90°	95°	100°	105°	110°	115°	120°
					Apparent Temperature*						
0%	64°	69°	73°	78°	83°	87°	91°	95°	99°	103°	107°
10%	65°	70°	75°	80°	85°	90°	95°	100°	105°	111°	116°
20%	66°	72°	77°	82°	87°	93°	99°	105°	112°	120°	130°
30%	67°	73°	78°	84°	90°	96°	104°	113°	123°	135°	148°
40%	68°	74°	79°	86°	93°	101°	110°	123°	137°	151°	
50%	69°	75°	81°	88°	96°	107°	120°	135°	150°		
60%	70°	76°	82°	90°	100°	114°	132°	149°			
70%	70°	77°	85°	93°	106°	124°	144°				
80%	71°	78°	86°	97°	113°	136°					
90%	71°	79°	88°	102°	122°						
100%	72°	80°	91°	108°							

HOW TO USE HEAT INDEX:
1. Across top locate Temperature
2. Down left side locate Relative Humidity
3. Follow across and down to find Apparent Temperature
4. Determine Heat Stress Risk on chart below

Apparent Temperature	Heat Stress Risk with Physical Activity and/or Prolonged Exposure
90°–105°	Heat cramps or heat exhaustion possible
105°–130°	Heat cramps or heat exhaustion likely Heatstroke possible
130° and up	Heatstroke highly likely

✔ **Note:** *Combined index of heat and humidity. . . what it feels like to the body.
✔ **Note:** This heat index chart is designed to provide general guidelines for assessing the potential severity of heat stress. Individual reactions to heat will vary. In addition, studies indicate that susceptibility to heat disorders tends to increase with age. Exposure to full sunshine can increase Heat Index values by up to 15°F.
■ **Source:** National Oceanic and Atmospheric Administration.

To reduce problems caused by heat and humidity, exercise at the coolest time of the day. Avoid practicing during the middle of the day when the temperature is usually the highest. If you must practice or compete then, gradually build up your tolerance to the heat by short workouts in the heat each day. Over time, the length of your workout can be slowly increased.

Clothing and sports gear also affect sweating and body temperature. Sweat suits and other heavy gear prevent evaporation and cause a buildup of body heat. Wear the lightest clothing possible in hot or humid weather. Mesh jerseys, lightweight shorts, and low-cut socks allow more heat to evaporate than do sweat suits and heavy gear.

HEAT ILLNESSES

Athletes who exercise in hot or humid weather can experience heat cramps, heat exhaustion, or heatstroke. Three factors contribute to the development of these heat injuries: increased body temperature, loss of body fluids, and loss of electrolytes.

Heat Cramps

Heat cramps (involuntary muscle spasms) occur during or after activity, usually in the specific muscles exercised. They are probably caused by imbalance of the body's fluid and electrolyte concentrations. Muscles spasms can occur if the electrolytes lost in sweat aren't replaced. The treatment is to rest, drink fluids with electrolytes (sports drinks), and add salt to foods.

Heat Exhaustion

Heat exhaustion may be caused by a reduced blood volume due to excessive sweating. Blood then pools in the extremities, and you may faint or feel dizzy. Symptoms also include nausea and fatigue. Although sweating may be reduced, the rectal temperature is not elevated to dangerous levels (less than 104°F). The treatment is to rest in a cool place and drink fluids containing electrolytes. Medical attention may be required.

Heatstroke

Heatstroke is a medical emergency requiring immediate action. The body's temperature-regulating processes simply stop functioning. Sweating usually stops, and the skin becomes dry and hot. The rectal temperature is excessively high—over 105.8°F. Other symptoms include disorientation, vomiting, headache, and unconsciousness. If heatstroke is untreated, death occurs due to circulatory collapse and central nervous system damage. The treatment is to immediately lower elevated body temperature. Until medical help arrives, the athlete can be covered with ice packs, immersed in cold water, or rubbed with alcohol.

Be aware of the symptoms of impending heat illness. These include weakness, a feeling of chills, goose pimples on the chest and upper arms, nausea, headache, faintness, disorientation, muscle cramping, and cessation of sweating. Continuing to exercise when experiencing any of these symptoms can lead to a heat injury.

FLUID REPLACEMENT GUIDELINES

At rest, you need at least 2 quarts or liters of fluid daily. Exercise greatly increases fluid requirements. Consuming fluids prior to exercise appears to reduce or delay the detrimental effects of dehydration. You should drink 17 ounces (500 milliliters) of fluid 2 hours prior to exercise. This promotes adequate hydration and allows time for the excretion of excess fluid.

Drinking during exercise is essential to prevent the detrimental effects of dehydration on body temperature and exercise performance. As shown in Table 9-2, you should drink 5 to 10 ounces (150 to 300 milliliters) of cool fluid every 15 to 20 minutes during exercise to replace sweat losses.

TABLE 9-2
Hydration Guidelines

- 17 ounces two hours before exercise
- 5 to 10 ounces every 15 to 20 minutes during exercise
- 24 ounces for each pound of body weight lost after exercise

---

The actual amount consumed during exercise will depend on your rate of sweat loss. However, there is no safe level of dehydration that you can tolerate before cardiovascular function and temperature regulation are impaired. You'll perform at your best when your fluid intake closely matches your fluid loss from sweating.

Thirst is not an adequate guide to fluid replacement. Most people replace only 50% of their fluid losses during exercise. Athletes need to regulate their fluid intake by drinking according to a time schedule rather than in response to thirst.

Get into the habit of regular drinking during training. Some athletes pay attention to their fluid intake only during competition and become dehydrated in practice sessions. Heat injury can occur just as easily during training. Adequate fluid intake during training protects against heat illness and enables you to get the most out of workouts. It also gives you the chance to practice proper hydration techniques for competition.

Occasionally, fluids are restricted during practice so that athletes won't "depend" on them during competition. This strategy doesn't make athletes better prepared for competition—it increases their risk of heat injury. The body can't adapt to becoming dehydrated.

Weigh both before and after exercise (nude is best) to determine how much fluid you're losing. You should drink 24 ounces of fluid (about 750 milliliters) for every pound of body weight lost. If you notice a gradual loss of weight during warm-weather training, this may be due to chronic dehydration rather than body fat loss. You can also check the volume, color, and odor of your urine. Urine that is of small volume, is dark yellow in color, and has a strong odor suggests that you are dehydrated.

FLUID-REPLACEMENT BEVERAGES

You can consume water or a sports drink to replace fluid losses. Sports drinks containing carbohydrate and sodium, such as Gatorade, are absorbed as quickly as water. The presence of glucose and sodium in sports drinks increases fluid uptake in the small intestine. Table 9-3 lists some popular sports drinks.

Sports drinks promote optimal cardiovascular function and temperature regulation as well as plain water does. However, unlike water, sports drinks improve performance during prolonged exercise by providing carbohydrate for the working muscles. For exercise lasting an hour or longer, sports drinks provide a performance edge that water can't. Sports drinks are also beneficial when you're exercising for an hour several times a day. Water remains an effective and inexpensive fluid-replacement beverage for exercise lasting less than an hour.

For optimal absorption and performance, a sports drink should contain 4–8% carbohydrate (10 to 18 grams per 8 ounces)—about 36 to 77 calories per 8 ounces. Beverages that exceed 10% carbohydrate (about 96 or more calories per 8 ounces), such as fruit juice and soda, take longer to be absorbed, as do drinks high in fructose. They can cause abdominal cramps, nausea, bloating, and diarrhea. Most sports drinks contain 5–8% carbohydrate.

Fluid-replacement beverages should be rapidly absorbed, taste good, and not cause gastrointestinal problems when consumed in large volumes. Beyond these concerns, it's a matter of personal preference. Try several different sports drinks during training to find the one that works the best for you.

ELECTROLYTES

Electrolytes such as sodium, potassium, and chloride are necessary for the maintenance of body fluid levels, muscle contractions, and nerve impulse transmission.

Sweating results in electrolyte losses (particularly sodium) as well as water losses. However, water losses during sweating are proportionately greater than electrolyte losses, so the body's cells end up with a greater electrolyte concentration. As you become acclimated to the heat, the sodium content of your sweat decreases.

Electrolyte needs can generally be met by consuming a balanced diet. Although sodium is the major electrolyte lost in sweat, our diets provide an abundance of salt (sodium chloride). The loss of 1 gram of sodium, which occurs with about a 2-pound sweat loss, can easily be replaced by moderate salting of food. One-half teaspoon of salt supplies 1 gram of sodium. Salt tablets should generally be avoided, as they can cause nausea by irritating the stomach lining and increase the body's water requirement.

Replacing potassium losses should not be a problem either. Athletes lose far more sodium than potassium during exercise. Orange juice, bananas, and potatoes are all excellent sources of potassium. A large glass of orange juice will replace the potassium lost in about 4 pounds of sweat. Potassium supplements are unnecessary and may be dangerous. They can cause an excessively high level of potassium in the blood, resulting in an abnormal heart rhythm.

Electrolyte deficits, particularly sodium, can occur under certain conditions—when acclimating to a hot environment, following repeated workouts in hot weather, and during ultra-endurance events such as 50-mile runs, 100-mile bicycle rides, and long triathlons (such as the Ironman).

Consuming only plain water during ultra-endurance events can cause a dangerous condition called hyponatremia (low blood

TABLE 9-3
Popular Sports Drinks

Ingredients per 8 oz.	Carbohydrate Content (%)	Carbohydrate (grams)	Carbohydrate Type	Calories	Sodium (mg)	Potassium (mg)	Carbonation	Caffeine
Gatorade Thirst Quencher GATORADE COMPANY	6%	14	Sucrose, Glucose, Fructose	50	110	30	No	No
AllSport PEPSICO, INC.	8%	20	High Fructose Corn Syrup	70	55–80	50	Yes	No
CeraSport CERA PRODUCTS, LLC	7%	16	Maltodextrin	76	102	37	No	No
Cytomax CYTOSPORT, INC.	6%	15	High Fructose Corn Syrup, Maltodextrin, Lactate	80	70	77	No	No
Met-Rx ORS MET-RX, INC.	8%	19	Fructose, Glucose	75	125	40	No	No
Metabolol Endurance CHAMPION NUTRITION	7%	16	Maltodextrin, Fructose	133	140	200	No	No
Powerade COCA-COLA COMPANY	8%	19	High Fructose Corn Syrup, Glucose Polymers	72	53	33	No	No
PowerBar Perform POWERBAR, INC.	7%	16	Glucose, Fructose, Maltodextrin	60	110	35	No	No

Ingredients per 8 oz.	Carbohydrate Content (%)	Carbohydrate (grams)	Carbohydrate Type	Calories	Sodium (mg)	Potassium (mg)	Carbonation	Caffeine
Pro-Hydrator INTERNUTRIA, INC.	0%	0	Glycerol is primary ingredient (no carbohydrate)	0	2.5	4.5	No	No
Revenge CHAMPION NUTRITION	4%	10	Maltodextrin, Fructose, Glucose	50	48	80	No	Yes
Ultima ULTIMA REPLENISHER	2%	4	Maltodextrin	16	8	16	No	No
NONSPORTS DRINKS								
Coca-Cola COCA-COLA COMPANY	11%	27	High Fructose Corn Syrup, Sucrose	100	35	0	Yes	Yes
Endurox PACIFIC HEALTH LABORATORIES	15%	35	Maltodextrin, Glucose, Fructose	187	180	93	No	No
Mountain Dew PEPSICO, INC.	13%	31	High Fructose Corn Syrup	110	50	0	Yes	Yes
Orange Juice	11%	27	Sucrose, Fructose, Glucose	112	7	446	No	No
Pedialyte ROSS LABORATORIES	2.5%	6	Glucose, Fructose	24	248	187	No	No
Rehydralyte ROSS LABORATOROES	2.5%	6	Glucose	24	407	183	No	No
Water	0%	0	None	0	0	0	No	No

sodium). Sodium losses in sweat during ultra-endurance events can be considerable, and consuming only water or low-sodium beverages dilutes the amount of sodium left in the blood.

Symptoms of low blood sodium include lethargy, muscle cramping, mental confusion, and seizures. Fortunately, this condition is rare (heat illnesses occur far more often) but can be fatal if untreated. You can reduce the risk of hyponatremia by consuming sports drinks that contain sodium.

Sports drinks containing sodium can also promote rehydration following exercise. The sodium helps to maintain thirst and keeps you drinking while it delays urine production. This promotes rapid rehydration and enhances recovery. Drinking plain water eliminates thirst so that you stop drinking and urine production is stimulated. This can delay rehydration and hinder recovery. In addition to aiding fluid absorption, the sodium in sports drinks encourages fluid intake because it makes the drink taste better.

ALCOHOL AND CAFFEINE

Consuming alcohol before or during exercise won't provide an energy boost and may harm performance. Alcohol is a central nervous system depressant that impairs judgment, reaction time, fine motor coordination (speech), and gross motor coordination (walking and balance). As mentioned in Chapter 2, excessive alcohol intake increases the risk of automobile accidents and causes numerous health problems.

Alcohol decreases the output of glucose by the liver, thereby causing low blood glucose levels and early fatigue. Alcohol may also contribute to hypothermia (dangerously low body temperature) during workouts in cold weather.

Even a bout of excessive drinking the night before exercise can hurt performance. Aside from the obvious adverse effects of the hangover—headache and nausea—heavy drinking causes

---

TABLE 9-4
Alcoholic Beverages

Beverage (% alcohol by volume)	Serving Size (oz)	Calories
Wine (11.5%)	5	105
Sherry (19%)	3	125
Beer (4.5%)	12	150
Stout or porter on tap (about 3%)	12	200
Gin, vodka, rum, whiskey (rye, Scotch), 80 proof (40%)	1.5	100–110
Cordials, liqueurs, 25–100 proof (12.5–50%)	1	50–100
Martini (38%, ¾ oz. alcohol)	2.5	156
Manhattan (37%)	2	128
Bloody Mary (12%)	5	116
Tom Collins (9%)	7.5	121
Daiquiri (28%)	2	111
Gin and tonic (9%)	7.5	171
Piña colada (12%)	4.5	262
Screwdriver (8%)	7	174
Tequila sunrise (14%)	5.5	189
Whiskey sour prepared from bottled mix (17%)	3.5	160

---

dehydration. The diuretic effect of alcohol may increase the risk of developing a heat illness during exercise in warm weather.

Since alcohol is a diuretic, you shouldn't use it to replace fluid losses immediately after exercise. The best post-exercise drink is one that contains carbohydrate and sodium to replace both glycogen and water.

The liver can get rid of only about a half-ounce of pure alcohol per hour—the amount found in one drink. A drink is equal to 12 ounces of beer, 5 ounces of wine, and 1½ ounces of 80 proof liquor. One or two drinks of this size daily appear to cause no harm to nonpregnant, healthy adult athletes who can afford the calories. Pregnant women should not drink since consumption of alcohol may cause birth defects or other problems during pregnancy.

Alcohol is a poor energy source because it doesn't contribute to the formation of muscle glycogen—the preferred fuel for most sports. One 12-ounce beer or 5-ounce glass of wine supplies only 50 calories of carbohydrate—enough to run a half-mile.

Alcoholic beverages are also high in calories and low in nutrients—a source of empty calories if you want to reduce your body fat. Substitute alcohol calories for fat calories—not food calories. Twelve ounces of beer provides 150 calories, while 5 ounces of wine or 1½ ounces of liquor each supply about 100 calories. Table 9-4 lists some common alcoholic beverages.

The caffeine found in coffee, tea, and some sodas is also a diuretic. If you drink caffeinated beverages, pay extra attention to your fluid intake at rest and during exercise. Diet caffeinated sodas, which are frequently chosen by weight-conscious athletes, are especially poor rehydration beverages because they increase urinary water losses.

10

BODY
COMPOSITION

In our society, the bathroom scale has a following worthy of a
political party or religion. An unbelievable number of
weight-loss gimmicks have been spawned by our obsession
with weight loss. In the rush to shed pounds, a very important
question is often overlooked: "How fat am I?"

The scale cannot differentiate between fat pounds and muscle pounds. The scale does not indicate how fat a person is,
because both fat and muscle, as well as bone and water, contribute to the total weight.

The term "overweight" refers only to body weight in excess
of the average for a specific height. The term "underweight"
refers only to the body weight below the average weight for
height. The scale is biased against stocky, muscular people, just
as it favors thin, slightly built people.

A more accurate indicator of fitness is body composition,
which divides weight into two categories. One is the fat-free
mass, of which muscle is a major component. The other category
is fat. What is really important is how much of a person's weight
is fat. This is expressed as **percent body fat**.

The person who suffers the most when evaluated by weight
alone is the stocky, muscular man or woman. Because these athletes

may have little fat, they weigh more than average because of a large fat-free mass. To lose weight, they may lose muscle and experience a deterioration in their performance and health. This is just one reason why body composition assessment is so important before trying to lose weight.

Athletes are somewhat restricted by their genetic inheritance. Body shape and size are largely determined by skeleton size, as a certain amount of muscle and tissue accompanies a certain amount of bone. Beyond heredity, your total amount and distribution of muscle mass will depend on the type of training you do. For example, weight training increases muscle mass more than distance running.

As athletes know, body type is important in most sports, and each sport seems to require a certain body type. The large, muscular person will never be an elite marathoner, just as an elite marathoner would not survive as an interior lineman on the football field.

While body size and shape can be altered only slightly, substantial changes can occur in body composition. These changes can significantly affect performance. In power sports, performance can be improved by extra muscle gained from weight lifting. It is also obvious that distance running can be harmed by excess body fat. However, athletes who train for a specific sport are likely to have the muscle mass that is appropriate for that sport. If, because of genetics, their muscle mass is greater than desired, they will only hurt themselves by trying to lose weight.

BODY FAT STANDARDS

A number of studies have been done to assess the body composition of athletes. The results suggest that body fat values differ widely both between sports and within sports. Thus, an ideal body fat for a particular sport is difficult to establish. Recommending a range for the percent body fat goal (5–8% body fat for a male marathon runner) is more appropriate than making a single point recommendation (5% body fat).

Before you attempt to achieve a certain percent body fat, there are several things to keep in mind. Success in a sport depends on a variety of factors. Having a low body fat does not, in itself, ensure you will be a superior athlete.

A healthy level of body fat for men is around 15%. A man who has 20% body fat is considered obese. A healthy level of body fat for women is around 25%. A woman who has 30% body fat is considered obese. The average range of body fat is 15–18% for men and 22–25% for women.

Three percent of the total body fat in men is considered "essential" fat. It appears that a man cannot reduce his body fat below this limit without impairing his physiological function and capacity for exercise.

The percentage of body fat considered "essential" for women is 12%. This higher level of fat is related to childbearing functions and takes into account sex-specific fat in the breasts, hips, and other tissues.

As an upper limit, try to be close to the healthy levels of 15% for men and 25% for women. Beyond this, your ideal percent body fat is where you perform the best.

Your weight and percent body fat should be monitored by a health professional and kept in a range that promotes your health and performance.

BODY COMPOSITION ASSESSMENT

The hydrostatic (underwater) weighing procedure involves weighing a person on a balance beam scale and then determining the weight of the person submerged under water. Since muscle is denser than fat (1 pound of muscle takes up the room of 1/3 pound of fat), people with more muscle and less fat weigh more under water. In other words, they have a higher body density and lower percent body fat.

Even though there are certain technical limitations to this procedure, hydrostatic weighing is referred to as the "gold standard" because it is the most accurate technique currently available to assess body composition. The standard error of measurement for hydrostatic weighing is about 2%. This means that an athlete with a "true" percent body fat of 15% may be measured as having 13%–17% body fat.

Anthropometry

Anthropometry consists of measurements of skinfold thicknesses, circumferences, and bone diameters. Measurements from different anatomical sites are used in mathematical equations to predict body density and percent body fat. These prediction equations are also usually validated against the "gold standard" of underwater weighing.

Like most clinical techniques of measuring body composition, anthropometry is indirect, which increases the measurement error. Just as with underwater weighing, percent body fat results obtained by anthropometry should be considered estimates— never absolute values.

Skinfold measurements are the most practical way to assess body composition. Skinfolds represent the thickness of a double layer of skin and the underlying subcutaneous fat, as determined by metal (not plastic) calipers. The rationale behind skinfolds is that about 50% of the total body fat is stored just under the skin as subcutaneous fat. Although less accurate than hydrostatic weighing, skinfold measurements are useful for determining regional distribution of subcutaneous fat in addition to estimating percent body fat. Also, combining skinfolds with circumferences can help to estimate muscle and bone changes.

Although procedures for taking skinfold measures are straightforward, the examiner must be properly trained in the specific anatomic skinfold sites (triceps, thigh, abdomen) and have had sufficient practice to take consistent measurements. Even in trained hands, skinfold measurement has a standard error of measurement of about 3–4%. This means that if an athlete's body fat is estimated to be 15%, it could be as low as 11% or as high as 19%.

Circumference, or girth, measures, when used alone or in combination with skinfold measures, help to evaluate fat patterning, muscular development, and frame size. Although the measurements appear easy to make, obtaining accurate readings can be challenging. Measures are taken with a plastic or metal tape measure at specific body sites such as the waist, hip, upper arm, or thigh.

The measurement of bone diameters (joint widths) is used to assess frame size and skeletal mass. Body weight varies with bone thickness, as well as with height and age. An individual with a greater bone weight has a greater body weight. Knowing frame size helps to distinguish those who are overweight due to a large fat-free mass (bone and muscle) and those whose extra weight is predominantly fat.

Bone diameters are measured with broad-blade anthropometers and small sliding calipers. Common sites selected for an estimation of frame size and skeletal mass are the elbow and wrist.

Other Methods

Bioelectrical impedance (BIA) involves passing a small electrical current throughout the body and measuring the resistance encountered through electrodes placed on the hands and feet. Lean tissue is a good conductor of electricity due to its high water content (about 70%), whereas fat is not due to its low water content (about 10%). The resistance encountered is inversely related to the amount of fat-free mass. Fat weight is then calculated by subtracting the fat-free mass from body weight.

BIA has become popularized (especially in health clubs) because it's an easy, quick, and noninvasive technique. Unfortunately, BIA tends to overestimate the body fat of a lean person and underestimate the body fat of an obese person. The method also assumes that the person is completely hydrated when the measure is taken.

Early research with impedance revealed large standard errors of measurement (about 7%), whereas newer techniques provide lower standard errors (3–4%) that are comparable to those of skinfold measurements.

Infrared interactance uses near-infrared spectroscopy to provide information about the chemical content of the body. The technique uses a fiber-optic probe that is pressed against the skin on top of the biceps muscle of the upper arm. A light beam is emitted that penetrates the subcutaneous fat and muscle, which is then reflected off the bone to a silicon detector in the probe. The procedure takes only 2–3 minutes to complete, and the subject is fully clothed. The standard error of measurement for this procedure is about 4–5%. Also, the validity of using a single site to represent the total body is questionable.

Both hydrostatic weighing and anthropometric measurements must be performed by trained personnel to ensure accuracy. This is why it is best to provide a range of desirable body fat values for an athlete.

CONSIDERATIONS FOR EVALUATING CHILDREN AND ADOLESCENTS

Evaluation in children and adolescents is complicated by several factors that affect the conceptual basis for estimating fat and lean tissue. Compared to adults, children have higher body water content and lower bone mineral content. This means their body density is lower than that of adults. Mathematical equations used for adults are not appropriate for children because they may overestimate body fat by 3–6% and underestimate lean tissue.

Another limitation is that the chemical composition of the fat-free mass changes as the child passes through puberty. Estimates of body fat by skinfolds, bone diameters, and circumferences may reflect alterations in the composition of the fat-free components (water, mineral, and protein) rather than alterations in actual fat content. Specialized equations have been developed that are appropriate for evaluating the body composition of children and adolescents.

Lastly, the body composition tables that show percent body fat values for male and female athletes are not suitable for children because most of these measurements were taken on older athletes. There are currently no standards of comparison for young athletes that are appropriate for sport and gender. The young athlete's weight and percent body fat should be monitored by a health professional and kept in a range that promotes optimal growth and development.

INAPPROPRIATE USE OF BODY WEIGHT/FAT STANDARDS

Body composition measurements are useful for monitoring changes in fat and lean tissue during training. When used inappropriately, however, the results can be disastrous. Attempting to reach an unrealistic percent body fat is as harmful as attempting to reach an unrealistic weight.

When an athlete's body weight or body fat drops below a certain level, both performance and health are adversely affected. Extreme weight loss can disrupt physiological function, nutritional status, hormone levels, bone mineral density, psychological function, and, for young athletes, growth rate.

Chronic fatigue often accompanies major weight loss. While the causes of this fatigue have not been established, both the central nervous system and endocrine system appear to be involved. Depleted fuel stores also probably play a role. When an athlete trains hard and consumes a diet that is inadequate in total calories or carbohydrate, muscle and liver glycogen stores become depleted. This causes weakness, fatigue, and impaired performance.

Fatigue may also result from the significant losses of muscle protein that occur when the body is forced to use protein for energy. Athletes who focus on maintaining an abnormally low body weight/fat during training often have inadequate intakes of vitamins and minerals as well.

Although body composition measurements are helpful in evaluating the fitness and performance of mature athletes, they should *never* be used in young athletes to manipulate body fat for sports participation or to set stringent weight-loss guidelines. Doing so may harm their growth and development.

11

LOSING FAT, GAINING MUSCLE

The energy that you obtain from food, as well as your body's energy expenditure, is measured in units of heat called kilocalories, abbreviated calories. Carbohydrate and protein supply 4 calories per gram, fat supplies 9 calories per gram, and alcohol supplies 7 calories per gram.

Weight loss, weight maintenance, or weight gain is a matter of energy balance. Your body weight will stay the same when your calorie intake equals your calorie expenditure. To lose weight, energy expenditure must be greater than energy intake. To gain weight, energy intake must be greater than energy expenditure. If you want to lose weight, you must eat less, exercise more, or do both.

Each person has a specific requirement for calories, determined by age, gender, body weight, and physical activity. The average adult female requires about 14 to 17 calories per pound of body weight daily, whereas the average adult male requires about 15 to 18 calories per pound daily. Physically active people, children, and adolescents require more calories per pound of body weight.

The calorie expenditure of your sport depends on the frequency, intensity, and duration of your activity. The more intense the exercise and the longer it's carried out, the greater the calorie expenditure.

You'll perform at your best if you achieve your competitive weight (while adequately hydrated) either in the off-season or early in the season. Allowing for an increase in lean tissue and decrease in body fat during training, try to maintain that weight throughout the season.

LOSING FAT THROUGH DIET

The National Heart, Lung, and Blood Institute has provided guidelines for promoting healthy weight loss. These guidelines indicate that the most successful strategies for weight loss are calorie reduction, increased physical activity, and behavior therapy designed to improve eating and activity habits.

The diet should be individually planned to help create a daily calorie deficit of 500 to 1,000 calories, depending on the person's calorie requirement. This moderate calorie restriction results in a reasonable loss of fat and minimizes loss of water, electrolytes, minerals, and muscle tissue. The initial objective is to reduce body weight by about 10% from baseline over a six-month period. The guidelines recommend a maximum weight loss of 2 pounds per week and suggest that ½ to 1 pound per week is optimum for most individuals (1 pound of fat equals 3,500 calories).

It helps to keep a diet diary to monitor food intake. This gives a good idea of how much and what you're eating to maintain your weight. After identifying where your calories come from, you can decide how to go about decreasing your intake. One way is to eat fewer "empty calories"—foods high in sugar, fat, and alcohol.

You can also cut calories by preparing smaller portions, using a smaller plate, eating more slowly, eating only fruit for snacks, reducing fried foods, and avoiding second helpings. The changes must be realistic for your lifestyle, since successful weight control requires a lifelong commitment.

Paying attention to calorie intake is critical for weight control. Some people think they can eat as much food as desired, as long as the food is fat-free. Consequently, they eat too many calories in the form of fat-free sweets and extra-large portions of starches. The result: They can't lose weight.

Cutting back on dietary fat does reduce total calories more than cutting back on carbohydrate, because fat supplies more than twice the calories by weight. Fat is also more likely to be stored as body fat than is carbohydrate. However, if you cut back on fat calories but add them back in the form of carbohydrate calories, you're not going to lose weight. It's a simple matter of energy balance that holds true whether you're an athlete or a couch potato.

LOSING FAT THROUGH EXERCISE

An effective weight-loss program incorporates both aerobic exercise (at least three days a week) and resistance training (at least twice a week) to reduce fat tissue and preserve lean (muscle) tissue. Athletes who don't expend many calories in their sport (gymnastics, baseball) can benefit by adding an aerobic exercise program to increase their calorie expenditure.

Aerobic exercise modestly decreases body weight and body fat, whereas fat-free mass remains constant or increases slightly. Resistance training significantly increases fat-free mass. This increases the resting metabolic rate because lean tissue requires more calories than fat tissue. By increasing the proportion of lean tissue to fat tissue, both aerobic exercise and resistance training increase the body's calorie-burning ability. These changes in body composition, along with the actual energy cost of exercising, help to create a calorie deficit and promote body fat loss.

Calorie restriction can dramatically decrease body weight and body fat, but also reduces lean tissue. When calorie restriction is combined with exercise, the loss in lean tissue is smaller than in programs using calorie restriction alone. Combining calorie restriction and exercise is the most successful way to enhance weight loss. In addition, individuals who combine exercise with calorie restriction are more effective in maintaining their weight loss.

To meet the threshold level for body weight and fat loss, you should exercise at least three days a week at a sufficient intensity and duration to expend 250 to 300 calories per session. An expenditure of at least 200 calories per session also promotes body weight and fat loss if you exercise at least four days per week.

In practical terms, 300 calories is roughly equal to walking 4 miles, jogging 3 miles, swimming 1 mile, bicycling 12 miles, or taking an aerobics class (including warmup and cooldown). As discussed in Chapter 7, the exercise intensity should be lower for an individual with a low initial level of fitness.

Increasing the frequency and duration of your exercise sessions will promote greater body fat loss due to a greater calorie expenditure. For example, you can burn off 2,000 calories each week by exercising four to five days per week and expending 400 to 500 calories per session.

GAINING MUSCLE

Increasing muscle mass can aid performance in strength and power sports. Body builders gain weight for aesthetic purposes. Ideally, you want to gain muscle rather than fat so that the new tissue can help your performance. An effective program to gain weight combines progressive resistance training (weight lifting) at least three times a week with an increased calorie intake.

You can generally gain about ½ to 1 pound of muscle each week. Since 1 pound of muscle contains about 3,500 calories, you must increase your calorie intake by about 500 calories per day to gain 1 pound in a week. You also have to add in the calorie cost of weight training (about 200 calories per hour workout). These calories are above and beyond the amount you normally require to maintain your body weight.

For example, if you require 2,500 calories per day and want to gain weight, you need an additional 500 calories per day to gain 1 pound of muscle per week. Add in your 200 calories per session of weight training (three times per week) for a total of 600 calories per week. When you figure in the extra calories for muscle gain and increased training, you require an additional 4,100 calories per week, or about 585 extra calories per day. This raises your calorie requirement to 3,085 calories per day.

Start by keeping a diet diary. This gives a good idea of how much and what you're eating to maintain your weight and how much more you need to eat to gain weight.

You can increase your calorie intake by eating larger servings of the foods you're currently eating (just the opposite of what is recommended for weight loss). It also helps to eat more often during the day by adding mid-morning, mid-afternoon, and bedtime snacks. You can drink commercial or homemade liquid meals with regular meals or as a snack between meals. The following suggestions may also help:

- Consume 1% or 2% fat milk instead of skim milk. Add low-fat cheeses to sandwiches or snacks. Eat fruit-flavored yogurt.
- Increase your intake of lean meat, poultry, and fish. Legumes are high in protein and low in fat. Use nuts, seeds, and small amounts of peanut butter for snacks.
- Eat more whole-grain products, such as breakfast cereals. Pasta and rice are nutritious side dishes. Quick breads and muffins can be supplemented with nuts and fruit.
- Add fruit to snacks and meals, and drink more fruit juices. Dried fruits such as apricots, dates, and raisins make excellent snacks.

- Eat fresh vegetables such as broccoli and cauliflower with melted low-fat cheese or low-fat sour cream dip. Increase your intake of starchy vegetables such as potatoes and corn.
- Fats have a high calorie density and so help to increase calorie intake. Use monounsaturated and polyunsaturated fats, and minimize intake of saturated fat.

You require about 1.6 to 1.7 grams of protein per kilogram when you're trying to build muscle. When you take in more calories, you take in more protein. As long as you consume enough calories, a diet supplying 12–15% of the calories from protein is adequate to increase muscle mass.

Since muscle is composed of about 70% water and 22% protein, 1 pound (454 grams) of muscle contains only about 100 grams of protein. To gain 1 pound of muscle a week represents an additional 14 grams of protein a day. This is easily supplied by 1 cup of nonfat milk and 1 ounce of chicken (15 grams total).

When your diet or supplements supply more amino acids than can be incorporated into new proteins, the excess amino acids are generally burned for energy. This causes excess urea production, which increases your body's water requirement as the body excretes the extra urea load.

UNHEALTHY WEIGHT-LOSS METHODS

While some weight-loss frauds merely slim down the wallet (instead of the body), others may endanger health and performance.

Low-Carbohydrate, High-Protein Diets

Many popular weight-loss books recommend a low-carbohydrate, high-protein diet. Carbohydrates are blamed for increasing the body's production of insulin and promoting body fat storage.

Low-carbohydrate diets cause a large initial loss of weight, primarily due to water losses associated with muscle and liver glycogen depletion. Without carbohydrates, the body doesn't burn fat efficiently and ketones accumulate in the blood. Ketosis suppresses the appetite but causes undesirable side effects such as nausea, headaches, fatigue, and bad breath.

In addition to ketosis, low-carbohydrate diets may cause dehydration, electrolyte loss, calcium depletion (due to high protein intake), fatigue (due to inadequate dietary carbohydrate), nausea (due to ketosis), gout, and possibly kidney problems. Inadequate intake of vitamins, minerals, phytochemicals, and fiber is also a concern on such unbalanced regimens.

What matters in weight loss isn't carbohydrates and insulin, but calories. Getting a high percentage of your calories from carbohydrate doesn't make you fat, because weight depends only on how many calories you take in relative to how many you burn off. High-protein, low-carbohydrate diets are not magic regimens —they're just very low-calorie. People lose weight on these diets because of the severe calorie restriction, not because of what is supposedly happening to insulin levels.

Athletes need adequate calories, carbohydrate, and fluid to perform at their best. Low-calorie, low-carbohydrate diets may harm performance by reducing muscle and liver glycogen stores. The dehydration and electrolyte losses associated with these diets may impair body temperature regulation and increase the risk of heat illnesses. And the symptoms of central nervous system depression that accompany ketosis—sluggishness, loss of coordination, inability to concentrate—are certainly not compatible with optimal performance.

Weight-Loss Pills

Nonprescription weight-loss pills, especially herbal products, are extremely popular. As with other dietary supplements, weight-loss pills are not regulated, so their ingredients and potency are not standardized. Many of these products combine the central nervous system stimulants ephedrine and caffeine, which supposedly increase energy and promote weight loss by raising the body's metabolic rate.

Ephedrine is structurally similar to the amphetamines and increases heart rate and blood pressure. Weight-loss products or herbs containing ephedrine (ma huang, Chinese ephedra, and *Sida cordifolia*) can cause serious adverse effects such as heart attack, stroke, seizure, psychosis, and death. The onset of symptoms such as dizziness, headache, gastrointestinal distress, irregular heartbeat, and heart palpitations following ephedrine ingestion indicates the potential for more serious adverse effects.

Side effects from ephedrine intake can vary and don't always depend on the dose consumed. These symptoms can occur in susceptible persons with low doses. There is also a question about potency, as the amount of ephedrine in the product may be higher or lower than the amount listed on the product label.

Caffeine is found in coffee, tea, some medications, and the herbs guarana and kola nut. Caffeine increases serum levels of epinephrine, thereby enhancing alertness and decreasing the perception of fatigue. Side effects of high caffeine consumption include nausea, muscle tremors, palpitations, and headache. Combinations of ephedrine and caffeine have side effects substantially greater than those from the consumption of either compound alone.

Athletes may not realize that ephedrine or other stimulants are in herbal weight-loss products because an unfamiliar herbal name for the stimulant is used. The unintentional use of such products may result in a doping suspension, since ephedrine is banned by the National Collegiate Athletic Association and the International Olympic Committee.

Many people assume that herbal weight-loss products are safe and without side effects because they are marketed as "natural" or "herbal" and can be purchased without a prescription. This belief that "natural equals safe" is common and can be a dangerous misconception. Some herbal weight-loss products even contain potent plant-derived laxatives (senna, cascara, aloe, buckthorn), diuretics, and other drugs that can cause abdominal cramps, nausea, fainting, breathing difficulties, fluctuation in body temperature, diarrhea, and even death.

Dehydration

Wearing rubber, plastic, or sweat suits during exercise in an effort to "melt away" fat is dangerous and ineffective. The weight loss is from fluid, not fat. The suit prevents the evaporation of sweat, which is necessary to reduce body temperature during exercise. This practice can cause dehydration, heat exhaustion, and even heatstroke. Lounging in saunas also causes weight loss from sweating. Of course, the weight will return to normal when the sweat-induced water loss is replaced.

Spot Reduction

Spot reduction to eliminate so-called cellulite from specific areas of the body is also vigorously promoted by creators of pills, creams, and "special" exercise equipment. The reality is that cellulite is simply subcutaneous fat that has a dimpled appearance. The only way to get rid of fat deposits is through diet and exercise. There is no way any cream, massage, or exercise can reduce fat on one part of the body.

Exercising a specific area does increase muscle tone and may make the person look thinner. For example, localized exercise such as sit-ups can cause substantial reductions in abdominal girth. This is not due to fat loss. Rather, the abdominal muscles are strengthened and are better able to hold in the abdomen.

Body wraps and elastic belts cannot "melt away" fat. They may appear to work by causing temporary water loss or tissue compression. Although the person may look thinner for a short time, only the wallet experiences permanent shrinkage.

EVALUATING WEIGHT LOSS PROGRAMS

"Miraculous" diets and products tend to produce only miraculous profits for their promoters. They are all based on the dream that a "magic" combination of foods and/or supplements can cause weight loss no matter how many calories are consumed. Believers are more likely to lose dollars than pounds.

All of these gimmicks can't be recommended for weight loss because they don't address eating habits, lifestyle, and metabolism. When evaluating a weight-loss program or product, consider the following points:

1. Does the diet include a variety of foods from the Food Guide Pyramid to ensure nutritional adequacy? Or does it suggest that a food or nutrient is either the "key" to weight loss or the primary "villain" that keeps people overweight? Be wary of diets that eliminate certain foods entirely or promote eating them in "special fat-burning combinations."

2. Does the program or product avoid sensational claims such as "quick and easy," "burns fat and builds muscle," "metabolically proven," "eat all you want and still lose weight," and "energizing"?

3. Is the diet's effectiveness well documented by research published in credible scientific journals (consult a registered dietitian) and not based on testimonials by famous people or self-proclaimed experts?

4. Does it call for behavior and lifestyle changes? Does it incorporate exercise?

5. Does it avoid the use of diuretics and/or appetite suppressants?

6. Does it consider the special sports-specific needs of athletes (fluids, calories, carbohydrates, protein, etc.)?

FOCUS ON BODY COMPOSITION

Body weight usually changes very little, if any, in the first few weeks of an exercise program. This is because lean (muscle) weight initially increases at about the same rate that fat weight is being lost. Individuals can become discouraged because the scales show no change, even though body composition (fat versus lean) is changing dramatically. During this time, people should pay more attention to how their clothing fits than what the scale says.

It is even possible to gain weight while losing fat (particularly when including resistance training) because of correspondingly greater muscle gain. For example, a person can gain four pounds of muscle but lose two pounds of fat. This often happens to sedentary women who begin exercising. They may drop two dress sizes but gain two pounds. Some have even quit exercising when this happens because they're conditioned to go by scale weight.

It's a good idea to have body composition evaluated before trying to lose or gain weight, and again periodically to measure any muscle gain and fat loss from exercise. Scale weight isn't an accurate indicator of body composition. And it can't give the real picture of the changes that can be expected from regular exercise.

12

NUTRITIONAL ERGOGENIC AIDS

"New performance breakthrough! Makes more energy available to your muscles. Increases your speed and strength without additional training. Our unique supplement is an energy-releasing substance extracted from natural foods by a secret process. Send $49.95 for your starter capsules now!"

But first, keep your hand on your wallet. If you're looking too hard for the magic bullet, you may find it in places it doesn't exist.

If you read a typical fitness magazine, you know there is no shortage of nutrition supplements that supposedly increase speed, enhance endurance, relieve muscle soreness, improve muscle mass, or reduce body fat. Some advertisements even claim their wonder product does all of the above.

All of us seek that "secret ingredient" that will enhance our workout and give us the edge over our competitors. As a result, we are susceptible to nutrition quackery—the promotion of false and/or unproved nutrition products and services for a profit. Quacks can be sincere and misguided individuals, as well as charlatans and frauds.

Quackery is successful because we want to believe in something magical that will improve performance more than hard training or prudent diet. In many events the difference between winning and losing is in divisions of seconds, so it is not surprising that we are vulnerable to miraculous claims for supplements.

The placebo effect by itself is powerful enough to produce beneficial results. When you are convinced that a supplement improves your performance, this belief may enable you to perform better, even though there is nothing useful in the product as such. Just because a friend may ride the placebo effect to a better performance, it doesn't mean that you will.

Most of the time, nutrition quackery only injures our wallet and creates false hope by promising impossible performance benefits. Quackery can, however, cause physical harm when necessary medical treatment for an injury or illness is delayed or abandoned.

PITCHES YOU SHOULDN'T CATCH

You can avoid being a victim of a nutrition rip-off by learning to recognize the techniques used to manipulate and deceive consumers. When you observe any of the following—stop, take a deep breath, and keep your money in your pocket.

The claims sound too good to be true, but they are what people want to hear. Nutrition quackery is successful because quacks play on emotions and misinformation. Most of us want to believe there are secret ways to improve our performance that can bypass the rigors of training and diet. However, we are rarely told of possible side effects or other harm that might result from the promoted product or dietary regimen.

Quacks also encourage distrust of reputable health professionals such as medical doctors, registered dietitians, and other nutrition scientists. They ridicule the nutrient content of our food supply and claim that the foods we need to meet nutritional requirements can't be purchased in grocery stores. They refer to their unproved treatments as true alternatives to reputable medical care. While choices do exist among current legitimate treatments, the alternatives promoted by quacks are usually ineffective and/or unsafe.

Quacks often use case histories, testimonials, and subjective evidence to justify their exaggerated claims. Quacks try to appear trustworthy by having well-known athletes promote their product. Testimonial evidence is by definition biased and uncertain. Scientists report their studies in reputable journals, where their work is reviewed and evaluated by other scientists prior to publication. Controlled experiments that can be confirmed by repeating the study are the best way to document the truth of the information.

EVALUATING CLAIMS

You need to be skeptical about the nutrition information you read and hear. Most victims of nutrition fraud aren't gullible, only unsuspecting. Magazines, books, and the media overflow with medical advice—some reliable and some inaccurate. Here are some guidelines you can use to evaluate nutrition claims:

- *What are the qualifications of the person recommending the product or diet?* A reputable person usually has a background or current affiliation with an accredited university or medical school offering programs in the fields of nutrition or medicine. Beware the title "nutritionist." It can be used by anyone, regardless of training. Even "Ph.D." is no guarantee. Sad to say, a quack can purchase the credential from a diploma mill (an unaccredited institution) to appear legitimate.
- *What evidence does the person supply for any claims that are made?* The claims should be supported with references to the scientific journals that published the original research. Is the information factual and specific, or vague and highly emotional? Are the recommendations based on published scientific evidence or on personal testimonials?

- *If the information is written, why was it published? Is someone trying to sell you something?* Does the material encourage gradual changes in your lifestyle, or does it promise to dramatically enhance performance or guarantee fast results? Does the author recommend eating a variety of foods, or are certain foods eliminated? Are expensive supplements recommended as the only way to ensure nutritional adequacy?
- *Do the suggestions appear to agree with most recommendations of medical and sports science professionals?* Professional journals review articles in a wide range of lay publications and judge their credibility. If you don't have access to these—and most athletes don't—you can seek the advice of a registered dietitian or other qualified nutrition professional at a local university, health department, or hospital. If you're considering big changes in eating habits that have kept you healthy until now, this extra digging is worthwhile.

ERGOGENIC AIDS

Nutritional ergogenic aids are dietary supplements that supposedly enhance performance above levels anticipated under normal conditions. The term *ergogenic* means "work producing."

Ergogenic aids generally have very little scientific evidence to back up their claims. Often, studies that are quoted to prove the product works haven't been published in respected journals or the findings of a study are misrepresented. Supportive research may also be poorly designed or use animals or human populations different from the populations buying the products.

Ads for such products often display muscular individuals and/or endorsements from body-building or weight-lifting champions. Locker room conversations about "bulking up" also perpetuate nutrition myths and misinformation.

Currently popular ergogenic aids (other than protein, amino acids, and vitamins) include the following:

- **Androstenedione** (an adrenal hormone that functions as a metabolic precursor to testosterone). *Claim:* Increases testosterone levels, increases muscle mass and strength. *Fact:* Little is known about the safety and effectiveness of androstenedione. It may be converted to testosterone in the body and produce muscle growth as do other illegal anabolic steroids. The known side effects of anabolic steroids include liver problems, unfavorable changes in blood lipids (decreased HDL and increased LDL), uncontrolled aggressive behavior ("roid rage"), increased acne, extra growth of body hair, reduction of testicle size and breast growth in men, and increased size of the clitoris and lowering of the voice in women. Anabolic steroids can also shut off bone growth in adolescents, stunting height. Androstenedione is banned by the NFL, NCAA, and Olympics.

- **Boron** (a trace element that influences calcium and magnesium metabolism). *Claim:* Increases serum testosterone levels, increases muscle growth and strength. *Fact:* These claims were based on a study which showed that boron supplementation increased estrogen and testosterone levels in postmenopausal women! The level of normal male testosterone is approximately ten times that observed in the study. At present, there is no evidence that boron increases testosterone levels, lean body mass, or strength.

- **Caffeine** (an alkaloid found in coffee, tea, and some medications that increases serum levels of epinephrine). *Claim:* Improves endurance. *Fact:* Consuming 3 to 6 milligrams of caffeine per kilogram one hour before exercise may improve endurance performance without raising urinary caffeine levels above the International Olympic Committee doping threshold. Although caffeine is a diuretic, none of the studies evaluating caffeine's metabolic and performance effects suggest that caffeine increases the risk of heat illness. Side effects of high caffeine consumption include nausea, muscle tremors, palpitations, and headache.

- **Carnitine** (a compound synthesized in the body from the amino acids lysine and methionine). *Claim:* Increases fat metabolism and decreases body fat. *Fact:* Carnitine facilitates the transfer of fatty acids into the mitochondria (the energy powerhouses of the cell) where they are burned for fuel in the aerobic energy system. There is no evidence that carnitine supplementation increases the use of fatty acids during exercise or decreases body fat. There is no dietary requirement for carnitine.

- **Choline** (precursor of the neurotransmitter acetylcholine and a component of lecithin, a substance involved in fat transport). *Claim:* Increases strength (by increasing acetylcholine) and decreases body fat (by increasing lecithin). *Fact:* There is no dietary requirement for this substance, and a deficiency has never been demonstrated in humans. The body can manufacture choline from methionine, an essential amino acid. There is no evidence that increasing choline intake will increase strength or decrease body fat.

- **Chromium** (an active component of the glucose tolerance factor, which facilitates the action of insulin). *Claim:* Increases muscle mass, decreases body fat, and promotes weight loss. *Fact:* Independent research by two USDA Human Nutrition Research Centers found that 200 micrograms of chromium picolinate daily and weight training for 8 to 12 weeks did not increase strength or muscle mass or decrease body fat. In November 1996, the Federal Trade Commission ordered the cessation of unsubstantiated weight-loss and health claims for chromium picolinate.

- **Coenzyme Q10** (a catalyst in the aerobic energy system). *Claim:* Optimizes ATP (adenosine triphosphate) production to increase energy and stamina. *Fact:* There is no dietary requirement for this substance, and a deficiency has never been demonstrated in humans. Supplementation with coenzyme Q10 does not improve endurance performance or maximum aerobic capacity.

- **Creatine** (combines with phosphate to form creatine phosphate, or CP, a high-energy compound stored in muscle). *Claim:* Increases CP content in muscles, improves high-power performance, increases fat-free mass. *Fact:* Research suggests that consuming 20 to 25 grams of creatine per day (5 grams consumed four to five times daily) for 5 to 7 days increases CP stores in trained subjects by 20%, delays fatigue during explosive sprint performance, and facilitates ATP resynthesis following sprint-type exercise. Short-term creatine supplementation increases strength and repetitive sprint performance by about 5–15% and body weight by about 2 pounds. Long-term creatine supplementation (the loading dose followed by 3 to 5 grams per day for several months) promotes significantly greater gains in muscular strength and repetitive sprint performance and increases body weight by about 7 pounds.

  Not all studies have found that creatine improves strength, sprint performance, or body weight. Creatine may not improve all high-power activities, since nearly all the studies have evaluated activities such as running, swimming, rowing, and cycling sprints, and weight lifting.

- **DHEA** (dehydroepiandrosterone—an adrenal hormone that functions as a metabolic precursor for the production of testosterone, estrogen, and other hormones). *Claim:* Increases testosterone levels, is a legal alternative to anabolic steroids, is an anti-aging hormone. *Fact:* DHEA is called the "steroid of youth" since levels decrease with age. There is no evidence that DHEA produces anabolic effects (e.g., increased muscle mass or strength) or decreased body fat in healthy, young adults. Side effects include oily skin, acne, extra growth of body hair, liver enlargement, and aggressiveness. The hormone's long-term safety has not been established, and, as with other hormones, adverse effects may not appear for years. Individuals who have a family history of breast or prostate cancer should not take DHEA. Mexican yam contains a plant sterol ring called diosgenin, which is a precursor for the semisynthetic production of DHEA and other steroid hormones, but this conversion takes place only in the laboratory.

- **Ephedrine** (a central nervous system stimulant and decongestant). *Claim:* Improves athletic performance, enhances weight loss. *Fact:* Ephedrine is effective for relieving bronchial asthma but is banned by the International Olympic Committee and National Collegiate Athletic Association. Ephedrine is structurally similar to the amphetamines and increases heart rate and blood pressure. Ephedrine-containing products can cause serious adverse effects such as heart attack, stroke, seizure, psychosis, and death. Combinations of ephedrine and caffeine have side effects substantially greater than those from the consumption of either compound alone.

- **Gamma-oryzanol** (a plant sterol derived from rice bran oil). *Claim:* Increases serum testosterone and growth hormone levels, increases muscle growth. *Fact:* Like other plant sterols, gamma oryzanol isn't ergogenic because it can't be converted to testosterone by the human body. It is poorly absorbed and appears to be safe.

- **Ginseng** (extract of ginseng root). *Claim:* Is an adaptogen (enhances immune system to increase resistance to stress and disease), improves performance, and a is "cure-all." *Fact:* Ginseng does not improve aerobic capacity or oxygen uptake. No other drug has all the healthful properties that are attributed to ginseng. The existence of a genuine cure-all is unlikely. Until proper research has been conducted, claims that ginseng has medicinal value should be considered unproved. Since ginseng root is expensive, the commercial preparations may contain little or no ginseng. The best-documented side effects of ginseng are insomnia and, to a lesser degree, diarrhea and skin eruption. The prolonged use of ginseng by adults seems to be relatively safe.

- **Glucosamine** (a naturally occurring aminosugar found in the building blocks of cartilage). *Claim:* Rebuilds cartilage, cures arthritis. *Fact:* In theory, supplemental glucosamine ensures rapid synthesis of cartilage, helping to overcome the degradation that occurs during joint diseases and cartilage diseases such as arthritis. There is some support for the efficacy and safety of glucosamine supplementation from both animal and human studies in the treatment of arthritis. Glucosamine salts are standard therapy for osteoarthritis in Europe. In the United States, preliminary research suggests that glucosamine sulfate may help early arthritis, but additional studies are required to confirm this.
- **Glutamine** (a nonessential amino acid). *Claim:* Enhances the immune system, decreases the risk of infection, helps to prevent the overtraining syndrome. *Fact:* Glutamine is a major energy source for gut enterocytes, lymphocytes, and brain cells, and it appears to be conditionally essential during times of metabolic stress and critical illness. Prolonged endurance exercise, such as the marathon, may reduce plasma glutamine concentration. Plasma glutamine concentration may also fall after periods of intense training that results in muscle glycogen depletion. However, an adequate daily intake of carbohydrate and other energy sources may help to prevent muscle glycogen depletion and overtraining as well as help to maintain normal glutamine status. Further research is required to determine whether glutamine enhances immune function in athletes.
- **Glycerol** (an alcohol that combines with fatty acids to form triglyceride). *Claim:* Improves thermoregulation and endurance performance. *Fact:* Glycerol hyperhydration may increase plasma volume and sweat rate, thereby reducing body temperature and improving performance during prolonged exercise in warm weather. Further research on glycerol's safety and efficacy is required.
- **HMB** (beta-hydroxy beta-methylbutyrate—a downstream metabolite of the essential amino acid leucine). *Claim:*

Increases muscle mass and strength, decreases muscle break-down after exercise. *Fact:* Supplementation with 1.5 to 3.0 grams of HMB daily during resistance training for three weeks may help increase muscle mass and strength. HMB may also protect against muscle damage during exercise or improve muscle repair following exercise. Further research is needed to confirm these findings.

- **Inosine** (a nucleoside involved in the formation of purines). *Claim:* Increases ATP production, increases strength, and enhances recovery. *Fact:* There are no research studies to support these claims for strength-trained athletes. Inosine may actually impair endurance performance.

- **Medium chain triglycerides, or MCTs** (fats which are water-soluble and readily absorbed). *Claim:* Promote muscularity and body fat loss, increase thermic effect. *Fact:* MCTs are ineffective as a fuel source during aerobic exercise. There is no proof that MCTs increase muscularity or enhance body fat loss in strength-trained athletes. Consuming large amounts can cause gastrointestinal upset and diarrhea.

- **Omega-3 fatty acids** (polyunsaturated fatty acids found mostly in fish oils). *Claim:* Stimulate release of growth hormone. *Fact:* Omega-3 fatty acids may be converted to prostagladins (hormone-like substances) in the body. A specific prostaglandin called PGE 1 may stimulate growth hormone release. However, there is no proof that omega-3 fatty acids improve endurance or strength.

- **Phosphates** (part of adenosine triphosphate, or ATP, and creatine phosphate, or CP). *Claim:* Improve endurance. *Fact:* Phosphate loading may increase intracellular phosphate levels and thereby increase oxidative metabolism. Phosphate loading may increase maximum aerobic capacity, blood lactate threshold and endurance. The dose is one gram of sodium phosphate, taken four times a day for three days. More research on phosphate loading is needed.

- **Pyruvate** (a three-carbon sugar produced at the end stages of the anaerobic energy system from the breakdown of glucose). *Claim:* Increases endurance, enhances fat loss. *Fact:* Consuming 25 grams of pyruvate and 75 grams of dihydroxyacetone, or DHA (another three-carbon sugar produced in the breakdown of glucose), for seven days improves both arm endurance and leg endurance in untrained men by 20%. The subjects experienced side effects in the form of intestinal gas and diarrhea. Obese, sedentary women who took 22 to 28 grams of pyruvate daily and ate only 500 to 1,000 calories for 21 days experienced greater weight and fat loss compared to the placebo group. The women who took pyruvate lost 37% (3.5 pounds) more body weight and 48% (2.9 pounds) more fat than the placebo group. The deceptively large percentage differences in weight loss amounted to only a couple of pounds. Keep in mind that commercial pyruvate preparations contain only 500 milligrams to 1 gram of pyruvate and may not contain DHA. Also, the subjects were untrained men or obese women, so pyruvate supplements may not help lean, active people. More research on pyruvate is warranted.
- **Smilax** (a genus of desert plants containing several species of sarsaparilla). *Claim:* Naturally increases serum testosterone levels, thereby increasing muscle growth and strength—a legal alternative to anabolic steroids. *Fact:* While Smilax does contain substances called saponins that can serve as precursors for the synthetic production of certain steroids, this conversion takes place only in the laboratory, not in the human body. There is no evidence that Smilax is anabolic or functions as a legal replacement for anabolic steroids. The saponins in Smilax have a strong diuretic action as well as some diaphoretic, expectorant, and laxative properties.
- **Sodium bicarbonate** (buffers lactic acid in the blood). *Claim:* Augments the body's buffer reserve, counteracts the buildup of lactic acid in the blood, and improves anaerobic performance. *Fact:* Several studies have supported improved anaerobic

performance (400- and 800-meter runs) with bicarbonate administration. Taking 0.3 gram per kilogram of sodium bicarbonate with water over a two- to three-hour period may improve 800-meter run time by several seconds. However, as many as half of those using sodium bicarbonate experience urgent diarrhea one hour after the soda loading is completed. The effects of repeated ingestion are unknown and caution is advised.

- **Vanadyl Sulfate** (a trace mineral with no dietary requirement). *Claim:* Promotes anabolic effects similar to those of insulin. *Fact:* Vanadyl sulfate has well-documented insulin-mimetic activity in non-insulin-dependent diabetes. A dose of 0.5 milligram per kilogram daily for 12 weeks did not increase strength or muscle mass during a weight-training program. Mild gastrointestinal symptoms and other side effects have been reported with vanadyl supplementation.

- **Vitamin B$_{12}$** (essential for DNA synthesis). *Claim:* Increases muscle growth and enhances strength. *Fact:* Since vitamin B$_{12}$ is essential for DNA synthesis, the theory is that vitamin B$_{12}$ or dibencobal (a coenzyme form of B$_{12}$) will stimulate muscle growth by enhancing DNA synthesis. However, there is no evidence that supplemental dibencobal or vitamin B$_{12}$ promotes muscle growth or enhances strength.

- **Yohimbine** (an alkaloid extracted from yohimbe bark that increases serum levels of norepinephrine). *Claim:* Increases serum testosterone levels, muscle growth, and strength and decreases body fat. *Fact:* There is no proof that yohimbine is anabolic. Tyramine-containing foods (red wine, liver, cheese) and nasal decongestants or diet aids containing phenylpropanolamine should be rigorously avoided when yohimbine is used to prevent a sudden and dangerous increase in blood pressure. People who have diabetes or cardiovascular, liver, or kidney disease should not take yohimbine.

REGULATORY PROBLEMS

The 1994 Dietary Supplement and Health Education Act bolstered sales by classifying dietary supplements in their own category and not as food additives or drugs. Dietary supplements are defined as vitamins, minerals, amino acids, and herbs or other botanicals.

Dietary supplements don't have to be proven safe or effective to be sold. There is also no guarantee that the product is what it says it is on the label. Whereas prescription and over-the-counter drugs and food additives must meet Food and Drug Administration (FDA) safety and effectiveness requirements, supplements that are marketed with medical claims bypass these regulations. These products can go to market with no testing for efficacy, thus skipping the years-long process that drugs must undergo.

The FDA is also prohibited from taking a product off the market unless the agency can prove that using the supplement will create a medical problem. Unfortunately, this law places the burden of proof of a supplement's safety on the overtaxed FDA rather than on the companies profiting from the sale of the supplement.

FDA approval is also not required for package or marketing claims. Although manufacturers of supplements are not supposed to make unsubstantiated health claims about their products, they easily get around this stipulation with the disclaimer "This statement has not been evaluated by the FDA. This product is not intended to diagnose, treat, or prevent disease." This disclaimer (usually in very small print) should raise a red flag of suspicion about the accuracy of the supplement manufacturer's information.

Lastly, supplements do not have to be manufactured according to any standards. Since supplements such as herbs are not regulated as drugs, no legal standard exists for their processing, harvesting, or packaging. In many cases contents, potency and purity are not accurately listed on the label.

THE BOTTOM LINE

New ergogenic aids for athletes are constantly emerging. Often, these products are marketed without any supportive scientific research to indicate their potential benefits or possible harmful side effects. Some products come on and go off the market before studies are done to establish or refute their claims. Prosecutions or other legal actions take years, and the promoter can reap huge profits during the delay.

Just about anything can be sold as long as it is called a dietary supplement. The 1994 Dietary Supplement and Health Education Act allows dietary supplements such as ergogenic aids to be marketed without proof of efficacy, safety, purity, or potency.

Your best protection against nutrition fraud is to be an informed consumer. If you have questions about a particular supplement, contact a registered dietitian specializing in sports nutrition.

13

EATING
ON
THE ROAD

O btaining a nutritious high-carbohydrate meal while traveling can be a challenge. Meal stops are often made at fast-
food restaurants because they are convenient and relatively
inexpensive. Although hunger may be satisfied, what about the
nutritional value of the meal? Did you get enough carbohydrate
to replenish glycogen stores? Did you eat too much fat? What
about vitamins and minerals? Lastly, did you drink enough fluids
for hydration?

No matter where you're traveling to compete, it is important
to choose foods that will fuel optimal performance. Finding
meals that are high in carbohydrate, moderate in protein, and
low in fat is the primary challenge. This chapter provides guidelines for making the best fast-food choices, strategies for choosing healthier meals at restaurants, tips for different cuisine, ideas
for meals and snacks at convenience and grocery stores, and air-
travel recommendations.

GOOD FOOD FAST

Although many fast foods are still high in fat and sodium
and relatively low in carbohydrate and fiber, food selections at

fast-food restaurants are constantly improving. Many offer
health-conscious options such as salad bars, prepared salads,
grilled or baked meat, fish or poultry, baked potatoes, low-fat
frozen yogurt or ice cream, and healthy soups. When nutritious
options are selected, fast food meals can be part of a healthy diet
and active lifestyle. You can use the general guidelines in Table
13-1 to help you make high-carbohydrate fast-food choices that
are moderate in protein and low in fat. Refer to Appendix A for
a detailed listing of high-carbohydrate, lower-fat fast-food
choices.

Breakfast

Simpler is better when it comes to fast-food breakfasts. Start
your day with cereal (hot or cold), bagels, English muffins, low-
fat muffins, pancakes, toast, fruit, and fruit juices. Add a scram-
bled egg and reduced-fat or skim milk or yogurt. Avoid breakfast
sandwiches made with cheese, sauce, bacon, or sausage, and side
dishes such as hash browns, Danish, croissants, and biscuits
because they are high in fat.

Lunch and Dinner.

Many fast-food chains offer high-carbohydrate, low-fat
lunch and dinner choices. Here's how to pick the healthier
options:

- *Burgers.* If you crave a burger, go for a single patty to keep
  fat intake to a minimum. Even two regular hamburgers have
  less fat than a double burger with cheese. Ask for extra
  tomatoes and lettuce, not sauce!
- *Chicken and fish.* Breading and deep fat-frying offsets the
  natural low-fat quality of plain chicken or fish. Order these
  foods grilled, roasted, or broiled, instead of fried. For flavor,
  add barbecue sauce or spices instead of a mayonnaise-based
  sauce.

TABLE 13-1
Making Lower-Fat, Nutritious Fast-Food Choices

Lower-Fat Choices	Moderate-Fat Choices	High-Fat Choices
Dairy Foods		
Low-fat milk	2% milk	Whole milk
Frozen yogurt	Soft-serve ice cream	Hard ice cream
Low-fat milk shakes	Milk shakes	
Starches		
Bagels, English muffins	Small order French fries	Biscuit, croissant
Pancakes, waffles	Cornbread	Hash browns
Cereals		Large order French fries
Bread sticks		Curly, cheese, or other fries
Baked potatoes		Pastry, pie, or brownie
Salad Bar		
Salad	Chicken, tuna salad	Olives, croutons
Carrot, celery sticks	Cole slaw	Bacon bits
Pasta	Macaroni/potato salad	More thsn 2 tbsp. dressing
Fresh fruit		Cream-based soups
Soups, not cream-based		
Low-fat dressings		
Meats/Main Dishes		
Chicken filet	Cheeseburgers	Fried chicken
Chicken fajita	Steak sandwiches	Fried chicken sandwich
Grilled chicken		Fried fish/fried fish sandwich
sandwich		Fish or chicken nuggets
Chili with beans		Super, deluxe, or supreme
Plain hamburgers		sandwich or burger
Vegetable pizza		Sausage, pepperoni, or extra
Chicken, turkey, ham,		cheese pizza
roast beef sandwich		Bacon burger
or sub		Breakfast biscuits (egg with
Bean burrito		sausage or steakk)
		Sausage, bacon
Sauces		
Catsup		Mayonnaise
Mustard		Mayo-type sauces
Barbecue sauce		Alfredo sauce
		Hollandaise sauce
		Added butter or margarine

- *Pizza.* Depending on the toppings, pizza can be a healthy snack or meal. Choose thin crust instead of thick-crust or deep-dish pizza. Choose vegetable pizza toppings such as mushrooms, spinach, onions, green and red peppers, hot peppers, pineapple, and broccoli to increase carbohydrate and reduce fat. Toppings such as extra cheese, pepperoni, and sausage add extra fat. For leaner protein options try chicken, Canadian bacon, or low-fat mozzarella or ricotta cheese.
- *Sandwiches.* Choose a regular or junior roast beef, chicken, turkey, ham and cheese (low fat if available), or vegetable sandwich. Tuna or chicken salad sandwiches made with regular mayonnaise will be higher in fat compared to ordering them plain. Instead of adding mayonnaise, oil, or special sauces, spice up your sandwich with oregano, pepper, mustard, barbecue sauce, low-fat sauces, tomatoes, vegetables, pickles, hot or sweet peppers. Order your sandwich on a roll, bagel, pita bread, tortilla, or hearty grain bread to increase carbohydrate and fiber. Remember, croissants and biscuits are not the best choice as they are high in fat.
- *Potatoes.* Have a baked potato topped with nonfat sour cream, chives, 2 tablespoons of grated cheese, mushrooms, broccoli, or chili. Avoid high-fat toppings such as cheese sauces, regular sour cream, and bacon. Go easy on French fries if you are trying to reduce calories and fat. Enjoy a small order of fries instead of a large order—or share a large with a friend!
- *Soup and salad bar.* When visiting the salad bar, choose salad greens, fresh fruits, vegetables, and plain pasta. Add lean protein to your salad with low-fat cheese, low-fat cottage cheese, kidney beans, egg whites, plain tuna, chicken, turkey, or roast beef. Pass on the prepared salads such as potato, macaroni, coleslaw, and pasta with mayonnaise or oil. Top your salad with raisins, croutons, chow mein noodles, and low-fat or

nonfat salad dressing. Soups such as chicken/turkey with noo-dles/rice, minestrone, vegetable, black bean, lentil, and green pea are healthy choices. In general, broth-based soups are preferable compared to cream soups, which supply significantly more calories from fat.

- *Southwestern.* Choose meals made with soft flour or corn tortillas instead of fried tortillas. Order quesadillas, soft tacos, or burritos made with chicken, beans, beef, or vegetables. Add low-fat condiments such as salsa, nonfat sour cream, lettuce, and tomatoes. Order a side of Mexican rice.

RESTAURANT STRATEGIES

Restaurant menus offer many clues to the fat content of foods. Words such as fried, crispy, breaded, scampi style, creamed, buttery, au gratin, and gravy all suggest that the food is high in fat. Better choices are items carrying such descriptions as steamed, broiled, boiled, charbroiled, poached, marinara, tomato sauce, and "in its own juice." Ask your server if you're not sure how a food is prepared based on the menu description. Most restaurants are willing to accommodate special requests such as low-fat or nonfat condiments, smaller portions, steamed vegetables, dressing on the side, and changes in food preparation to reduce fat content of the meal. Some restaurants include lower-calorie or heart-healthy fare on the menu.

TIPS FOR DIFFERENT CUISINE

Chinese

When dining at Chinese establishments, choose stir-fried dishes along with steamed rice and vegetables. Avoid deep-fried items (egg rolls and wontons) and high-fat foods such as spareribs and sweet and sour pork/shrimp. Fried chow mein noodles, fried rice, egg rolls, and lobster sauce (made with egg yolks) are "hidden" sources of fat. Some Chinese food choices with less fat are steamed rice; chicken chow mein; chicken/beef chop suey; steamed Chinese vegetables; stir-fry with shrimp, vegetable, chicken, Hunan tofu; hot-and-sour soup, wonton soup; fortune cookies.

Indian

Foods from India feature beans, rice, grains, vegetables, and bread, all of which are high in carbohydrate and low in fat. The food is often steamed, thus adding little fat. Dishes made with coconut milk and cream contain saturated fats and should be consumed in limited quantities.

Italian

At Italian restaurants, pasta is a good choice, but marinara sauce is recommended over alfredo and pesto sauces, which are high in fat. Thick-crust plain cheese or vegetable pizza is another good choice, as are salads with dressing on the side. Choose bread or bread sticks and limit butter, margarine, and olive oil. Some lower-fat Italian choices are pasta with marinara, tomato sauce, red clam sauce, chicken marsala, spinach or mushroom tortellini, minestrone soup, and Italian ice.

Mexican

At Mexican restaurants, chicken and bean burritos (not deep fried), soft tacos, and tostados are good choices. When available, pot beans or black beans can be substituted for refried beans. (Some restaurants offer refried beans that are fat-free or made with vegetable oil instead of lard—ask your server). Heated corn tortillas can be substituted for chips, and salsa can be substituted for sour cream (or ask for low-fat) and guacamole, which is also high in fat. Mexican food choices that are lower in fat include salsa, baked tortilla chips, gazpacho soup, black beans, red beans, Spanish rice, fajitas, chicken or seafood tacos made with flour or corn, and refried beans made without lard.

GROCERY AND CONVENIENCE STORES

If you're on a tight budget or looking for more options, a grocery store can offer a variety of high-carbohydrate, low-fat foods—even a soup and salad bar. Many athletes stop at convenience stores for snacks while traveling. Which snacks are high in carbohydrate and low in fat? For information on specific snacks, always check the food label. As a general guideline, a snack that contains at least 4 grams of carbohydrate for every 1 gram of fat will fall into the category of being a high-carbohydrate, low-fat snack. Let's take a stroll through a grocery store to evaluate some typical snacks.

A 2-ounce bag of potato chips offers 306 calories, but 58% come from fat and only 38% from carbohydrate. By comparison, a 2-ounce bag of corn chips has about the same amount of calories, but 43% come from carbohydrate and 51% from fat— less fat than potato chips but still higher in fat than recommended. Don't be fooled by chips disguised as fruit—1 ounce of banana chips provides 147 calories with 58% from fat and 44% from carbohydrate! To obtain savory snack choices low in fat, select pretzels (1 ounce has 108 calories with 83% from carbohydrate and 8% from fat), air-popped popcorn (3.5 cups has 108 calories with 82% from carbohydrate and 10% from fat), fat-free granola bars and fat-free breakfast bars (at least 95% of calories as carbohydrate), and rice cakes (21 calories each, with 88% from carbohydrate).

Nuts and seeds, though full of nutrients, are even higher in fat and calories than chips. Peanut butter supplies 95 calories per tablespoon—with 78% of calories from fat. Two ounces of roasted peanuts provides 344 calories. A whopping 73% of these are fat calories, while only 15% are carbohydrate. Likewise, 2 ounces of almonds translates into 352 calories, 83% from fat and 13% from carbohydrate. Be wary of snacking on sunflower seeds: Two ounces provides 314 calories, 76% from fat and 14% from carbohydrate.

Cookies provide lots of calories, primarily from fat and sugar. For example, two large Pepperidge Farm chocolate chip cookies provide about 320 calories, of which 55% are carbohydrate but 41% are fat. Two large Pepperidge Farm oatmeal cookies provide 305 calories, of which 58% are carbohydrate and 38% are fat.

Fig bars are a lower-fat selection. Two provide only 106 calories, 80% from carbohydrate and just 17% from fat. Because their calorie content is lower than that of most cookies, they're a good sweet snack choice for calorie-conscious athletes. Fat-free cookies, such as Snack-Wells, provide carbohydrate calories, but not fat calories.

Candy bars are a favorite snack choice. A Snickers provides 270 calories, 43% from fat and 49% from carbohydrate. Most candy bars contain about an equal proportion of fat and carbohydrate. Milky Way and York Peppermint Pattie are exceptions: Of the 260 calories in a Milky Way bar, 66% are from carbohydrate and 31% are from fat. A York Peppermint Pattie has 180 calories, 76% from carbohydrate and 20% from fat. Hard candies, jelly beans, gummy bears, candy corn, and licorice provide mainly carbohydrate calories and little or no fat. Table 13-2 lists some low-fat, high-carbohydrate candy.

Most pastry items contain more fat than carbohydrate due to added fat in frying or in fillings. For instance, a Hostess cake donut provides 115 calories, of which 44% are carbohydrate and 55% are fat. A regular raspberry Danish twist provides 220 calories—49% from fat and 49% from carbohydrate—compared to a fat-free raspberry Danish twist that has 140 calories, none from fat and 94% from carbohydrate.

TABLE 13-2
Low-Fat, High-Carbohydrate Candy

Food Item	Serving Size	KCAL	Carbohydrate	Fat
Bit-O-Honey	1.7 oz.	200	78%	18%
Butterscotch (Brach's)	3 pieces (0.6 oz.)	70	97%	0%
Candy corn (Brach's)	21 pieces (1.4 oz.)	150	99%	0%
Caramels	2 pieces	60	80%	20%
Jelly beans (Brach's)	12 pieces (1.4 oz)	140	100%	0%
Gummy bears (Brach's)	5 pieces (1.4 oz)	130	99%	0%
Fruit Juicers (Life Savers)	2	80	100%	0%
Peanut brittle (Kraft)	1 oz.	130	62%	34%
Peanut chews (Goldenbera's)	4 pieces (1.7 oz.)	215	60%	29%
Skittles	1.5 oz.	170	89%	11%
Starburst	8 pieces (1.4 oz)	160	83%	17%
Twizzlers	4 pieces (1.4 oz)	130	93%	7%
York Peppermint Pattie	1 (1.5 oz.)	180	76%	20%

The bread aisle provides foods that are low-fat and packed with complex carbohydrates and B-vitamins. Try bagels, whole-grain rolls and breads, raisin bread, English muffins, soft pretzels, and pita bread. Try cereals such as Raisin Bran, Chex, Wheaties, Cheerios, and cornflakes.

While regular ice cream is high in fat, there are nonfat or low-fat ice creams, sorbets, and frozen yogurt. For example, whereas a Dove Bar provides 350 calories and 51% fat, an ice-cream sandwich supplies 167 calories, 62% from carbohydrate and only a third from fat. A popsicle or juice bar has no fat —all of its calories come from carbohydrate in the form of sugar.

Probably the best selection in the dairy aisle is yogurt. A cup of fruit-flavored low-fat yogurt is 225 calories, of which 75% come from carbohydrate and only 10% from fat. Low-fat or fat-free pudding and yogurt are also available and provide fewer than 225 calories, with carbohydrate and protein. Unlike ice cream, fruit bars, and popsicles, yogurt is nutrient-dense with calcium, protein, and B vitamins. Low-fat cheeses and low-fat or nonfat milk are other healthy dairy snacks.

It's easy to find high-carbohydrate items in the cold drinks section. A twelve-ounce soda supplies 140 to 180 calories, all of which are carbohydrate in the form of sugar. A more nutritious carbohydrate alternative that's also 100% carbohydrate is fruit juice, which supplies, on average, 180 calories per 12 ounces. Other good choices are sports drinks containing 4–8% carbohy-drate (about 36 to 77 calories per 8 ounces). If the goal is rapid replacement of fluid loss, a sports drink is the beverage of choice instead of juices and soda, because the sports drink is better for-mulated to replenish body fluids rapidly.

Fresh fruit is another healthy choice. Fruit is nearly 100% carbohydrate and supplies vitamins, minerals, and fiber. A banana provides about 120 calories and an apple and orange each supply about 60.

AIR TRAVEL

Air travel presents some unique challenges. The pressuriza-tion of the cabin increases fluid losses, so dehydration can be a problem when the flight lasts several hours or longer. In fact, dehy-dration is thought to contribute to jet lag. Consuming beverages containing alcohol and caffeine increases the risk of dehydration because of the diuretic nature of these beverages. During air travel emphasize nondiuretic fluids such as water, sports drinks, and fruit juices to replace fluid loss.

Airlines don't always provide low-fat meals. However, low-fat or vegetarian meals are often available when requested in advance. You can also pack high-carbohydrate, low-fat snacks. If a meal is not provided on the plane, airport concession stands provide some healthy snacks and meals such as soft pretzels, popcorn (without butter), bagels, fruit/vegetable plates, juice, and frozen yogurt. At most airports, family-style and fast-food restaurants are usually available.

Depending on the destination, most athletes who travel internationally have difficulty finding enough food and familiar foods, and they are concerned about foodborne illness. Athletes who travel have a 50% chance of contracting travelers' diarrhea that sometimes requires medical attention and typically causes discomfort, concern, and dehydration. Bacterial infection of the intestinal tract occurs because of inadequate health standards for food and water in some countries, and because athletes have not had the chance to develop immunity to the pathogens in the places where they are competing.

Precautionary measures can be taken to protect against disease-causing organisms not found at home. Some suggestions are to drink only bottled water (even if brushing teeth); avoid swallowing shower water; not use ice cubes made from the local water supply; get restaurant recommendations from the U.S. Embassy, hotel managers, and coaches and athletes who have been in the area previously; stick to familiar foods; choose well-cooked foods; avoid milk and milk products because they require pasteurization and refrigeration; eat fruit that can be peeled (bananas, oranges, grapefruits, mangoes, kiwi); avoid salads and other uncooked foods that come in direct contact with the hands of the kitchen staff. It is advisable to pack foods to take along. Suggestions for nonperishable items include

- bread sticks
- high-carbohydrate beverages
- canned fruit/fruit juices, tuna, chicken, soups, baked beans
- cold cereals
- crackers
- dried fruit
- fig bars
- granola and breakfast bars
- sports nutrition shakes
- oatmeal
- peanut butter and jelly
- popcorn (microwave)
- pretzels
- pre-packed puddings, Jell-O
- sports drinks
- water (bottled)

Planning is key to finding high-performance fuel choices at fast-food franchises, restaurants, and grocery stores. Air travel poses additional challenges when you are striving to maintain a training diet that is high in carbohydrate and fluids, moderate in protein, and low in fat.

14

EATING DISORDERS: THE SILENT DILEMMA

Women are vulnerable to a variety of social, economic, and emotional stigmas associated with their weight. It is difficult to feel good about oneself in a society that rewards thinness and scorns people who are overweight—particularly when the overweight person is a woman. Under the influence of this strong cultural bias for thinness, many women are unhappy with their body size and shape, believing that they are never thin enough. This fear of fatness drives large numbers of women to live their lives on a continuous quest to lose weight.

The constant struggle to control weight can cause many women, particularly active ones, to engage in a variety of disordered eating patterns. At the very least, a woman's disrupted body image and disordered eating behavior perpetuates ongoing feelings of failure and poor self-esteem.

Many female athletes and active women believe that restricting their food intake will help them train and perform better, in addition to enhancing their overall appearance. Actually, restricting food intake can cause depleted energy stores, muscle wasting, weakness, fatigue, stress fractures, and impaired performance. Although some women manage to exercise and perform well for a while without an obvious decline, injuries and lack of energy will eventually take a toll.

PREVALENCE

Female athletes are at greater risk for eating disorders than are female non-athletes or males. Eating disorders can occur in any sport—or at any level of physical activity or fitness. However, they appear to be more prevalent in sports where appearance is judged (gymnastics, figure skating, diving, ballet, and body building), in weight-classification sports (wrestling, lightweight crew, and jockeys), and in sports that emphasize leanness to enhance performance (distance running and swimming).

While self-reports are generally used to establish the prevalence of eating disorders, the usefulness of this method is questionable. Even when anonymity is guaranteed, athletes may be reluctant to respond truthfully for fear they'll be discovered, labeled, or lose their position on the team. This may explain why some studies show increased levels of eating problems and others do not.

The prevalence of eating disorders may be as high as 50% in the sports noted above. Although 90% of eating disorders occur in females, 10% occur in males. Recognition and treatment of eating disorders in men can be difficult, due to the misconception that men are not affected by eating disorders and body image issues.

It's important to note that athletes in high-risk sports may have weight loss and dietary behaviors similar to those with eating disorders. A health professional is needed to distinguish between behaviors that may be associated with sports-induced requirements and the existence of an actual eating disorder. Recognizing the signs of eating disorders helps to facilitate early identification and treatment.

DEFINITIONS AND DIAGNOSTIC CRITERIA

Although recognition of these life-threatening disorders in athletes is growing, appropriate intervention and treatment lag far behind the problem. The revised fourth edition of the *Diagnostic and Statistical Manual of Mental Disorders* (DSM-IV-R), American Psychiatric Association (1994), defines eating disorders as severe disturbances in eating behavior. The diagnostic criteria for these disorders are defined below.

- *Anorexia nervosa* is characterized by refusal to maintain body weight at or above a minimally normal weight for age and height (less than 85% of that expected), a distorted body image (the person "feels fat" even when emaciated), an intense fear of gaining weight or becoming fat while being underweight, and amenorrhea (the absence of at least three consecutive menstrual cycles). Individuals with anorexia nervosa may be the binge-eating/purging type or the restrictive type who does not binge or purge.
- *Bulimia nervosa* is characterized by binge eating (rapid consumption of large amounts of food in a short period of time and lack of control over eating during the episode) followed by inappropriate compensatory behavior to prevent weight gain, such as self-induced vomiting, misuse of laxatives, diuretics, or enemas, fasting, or excessive exercise. The binge eating and inappropriate compensatory behaviors both occur at least twice a week for at least 3 months, and self-evaluation is unduly influenced by body shape and weight.
- *Eating disorder not otherwise specified* (NOS) describes disorders that do not meet the criteria for a specific eating disorder. Examples of NOS include individuals who binge-eat infrequently and individuals who have all the features of anorexia nervosa but have regular menses or a normal body weight.

The term *anorexia athletica* is used to identify athletes who show significant symptoms of eating disorders but who do not meet the DSM-IV-R criteria for anorexia nervosa, bulimia nervosa, or NOS. The classic features of anorexia athletica are an intense fear of weight gain or becoming fat even though the individual is lean, weight loss accomplished by a reduction in energy intake (often combined with exercise), and restrictive energy intake below that required to maintain high training volume. Binge eating is common, and such athletes frequently use pathogenic methods of weight control such as vomiting, laxatives, and diuretics. Some athletes with anorexia athletica also meet the criteria of NOS.

RISK FACTORS FOR EATING DISORDERS IN ATHLETES

Why are athletes at a greater risk for developing eating disorders? To answer this question, it is important to appreciate the many sport-specific expectations, performance demands, and other factors that influence athletes. An understanding of these can help to facilitate early identification and treatment.

Cultural Factors

Adolescents, especially women, are faced with enormous pressure to be thin and have an aesthetically pleasing appearance. Young women are continually bombarded with the message via fashion magazines and the media that having the "perfect body" symbolizes success, self-control, mastery, acceptance, and other values which are highly regarded by society.

For the adolescent female, changes in body composition (such as increased body fat) may be disconcerting even though this is a natural part of the maturation process. The inability to control weight and body shape may lead to a sense of frustration, guilt, and despair. Sports-related pressures and expectations go beyond the physical and emotional challenges already faced by athletes, particularly adolescent females. These stressors may initiate the development of a pattern of unhealthy eating that sets the stage for an eating disorder.

Psychological Factors

The behavior and attitudes of individuals with eating disorders and some athletes can overlap. Although high self-expectation, persistence, independence, perfectionism, competitiveness, and being goal-oriented may lead to excellence in the athletic arena, these qualities may also set the stage for an eating disorder. When an athlete with a vulnerable predisposition initiates a rigorous diet to manipulate body weight, it may become a self-perpetuating, self-reinforcing process.

Attraction to Sports and Exercise

Participation in certain sports may attract individuals who already have characteristics of eating disorders, at least in personality and attitude if not in behavior or weight. For the eating-disordered athlete, abnormal eating and dieting behavior can be hidden or legitimized through sports. The athlete may try to "blend in" with others who are trying to meet the stereotyped standards of body shape in certain disciplines.

Competitive Status

It is not clear whether elite athletes are at greater risk than nonelite athletes. It can be argued that risk factors such as perfectionism and fear of failure may be more pronounced among elite athletes, increasing the risk for an eating problem. Or, in athletes attempting to become elite, other pressures escalate and extreme measures may be taken to reach a higher goal.

Does exercise induce eating disorders? It has been theorized that intense exercise suppresses appetite. As a result, food consumption decreases and body weight is reduced. As weight decreases further, the drive for more exercise increases. Although this theory has some support, not all individuals with anorexia nervosa exercise, and this theory does not explain bulimia nervosa.

Early Training

Having a certain body type may steer an individual toward a particular sport. For example, an adolescent who is tall and has a large frame would be more likely to opt for volleyball or basketball where height and size are viewed as an advantage, rather than gymnastics where short stature and leanness are beneficial. Depending on the sport, the more the athlete's body deviates from the perceived ideal weight and body type, the higher the risk for an eating problem as the athlete struggles to meet the "ideal."

Athletes with eating disorders have been shown to begin sport-specific training significantly earlier than athletes who don't have eating disorders. Early training before maturity may prevent an athlete from choosing a sport more naturally suited to adult body type. However, in sports where thinness is emphasized (e.g., gymnastics and figure skating), there is a strong trend toward an ever-younger group of athletes who may complete their amateur career prior to puberty or shortly thereafter.

Dieting and Weight Fluctuation

Periods of restrictive dieting and weight fluctuation have been suggested as a risk factor or trigger for the development of eating disorders. Weight fluctuation may occur during the competitive season. For example, some athletes routinely struggle to achieve a low weight before competition, only to gain weight afterward when restraint weakens or other physiological processes promote restoration of a natural higher body weight. Weight change can be dramatic—some athletes lose and regain 10 to 15 pounds every week. Other athletes cycle between seasons. By using food and fluid restriction and exercise, the athlete keeps weight consistently below typical off-season body weight for the competitive season. Weight is regained to typical weight during the off-season.

Injury, Illness, or Loss of Coach

Some athletes have shown dramatic weight loss after losing or changing a coach, or following unexpected illness or injury. These circumstances may be viewed by athletes as a threat to continued success in their sport and may trigger an eating problem. Sexual abuse has also been reported as another possible explanation for the development of eating disorders among females. Unfortunately, there are documented cases of abusive relationships between male coaches and female athletes.

Athletes who have a fear of failure or performance anxiety may use an injury or a decline in performance related to an eating disorder to justify disqualification or dismissal from the team.

Weight Expectations: Coaches, Trainers, Parents

Dieting has been shown to act as a trigger for extreme weight loss. However, if the athlete receives guidance on how to lose weight, the risk of developing an eating problem may be minimized.

Pressure to reduce weight by coaches has been proposed as an explanation for the development of some eating disorders among athletes. Inappropriate and insensitive comments such as "you look fat," "you're a pudge ball," or "you could lose a few" which are often made to "motivate" the athlete may trigger an excessive response in an individual who is susceptible to an eating disorder. Similar misunderstanding or weight-related demands may also come from family, friends, or teammates.

RECOGNITION OF EATING DISORDERS

Often, the early signs and symptoms of eating disorders are ignored until the situation becomes serious. Although it is difficult to talk to someone about the possible presence of an eating disorder, ignoring the problem only increases the danger to the person. Seeking outside assistance from health professionals (physician, psychiatrist, psychologist, nutritionist) to discuss the person's problem (in confidence) can be reassuring and help define treatment alternatives.

Unusual eating patterns or behaviors may come to the attention of health professionals, coaches, friends, or parents through concerned team members who have noticed symptoms in a teammate. The coach may also observe decrements in performance and erroneously attribute them to a lack of effort or concentration. Whereas excessive weight loss is the most prominent clue to the recognition of anorexia nervosa, the athlete suffering from bulimia nervosa can appear healthy. Recognition of the problem may occur only with discovery of the associated behaviors of bingeing and purging.

Key symptoms of eating disorders are presented in Table 14-1. These symptoms do not in themselves signify that an eating disorder exists, but several signs justify the need for further examination by a health professional. Coaches and trainers should use the following guidelines when faced with a suspected eating disorder in an athlete. (Adapted from Rosen and colleagues, *The Physician and Sports Medicine*, 1986; 14: 79–86.)

1. Arrange a private meeting with the athlete. Under no circumstances should the athlete be spoken to about eating behaviors in front of a teammate.
2. Be direct and supportive in stating your concern. Tell the athlete specifically what behaviors/symptoms led you to think there is a problem.
3. Make certain the athlete understands that the discussion is confidential.
4. State your concerns for that athlete as a person—not as the star player on the team. Health and well-being take precedence over her or his role as an athlete.
5. Address any concerns the athlete has about the eating disorder affecting sports participation. Reassure the athlete that

---

TABLE 14-1
Physical and Behavioral Features of Eating Disorders

PHYSICAL FEATURES

- Weight too low for athletic performance
- Precipitous weight loss
- Extreme fluctuations in weight
- Bloating or edema
- Swollen salivary glands, puffy cheeks, or jaw just in front of ear
- Amenorrhea
- Proclivity to stress fractures
- Loss or thinning of hair
- Sores or calluses on knuckles or back of hand from induced vomiting
- Muscle cramps
- Gastrointestinal complaints
- Headaches, dizziness, weakness due to electrolyte disturbances
- Numbness, tingling in limbs

BEHAVIORAL FEATURES

- Excessive dieting
- Excessive eating without weight gain
- Excessive exercise that is not part of the training program
- Guilt about eating
- Claiming to feel fat at normal weight
- Preoccupation with food, calories, and weight
- Denial of hunger
- Hoarding food
- Frequent weighing
- Evidence of binge eating—food wrappings, etc.
- Likely self-induced vomiting—bathroom visits just after heavy meals, etc.
- Use of drugs to control weight—laxatives, diet pills, diuretics, emetics
- Mood swings
- Avoiding food-related social activities
- Relentless, excessive exercise
- Wearing baggy, layered clothing

Source: Adapted from D.M. Garner and L.W. Rosen,
J. Appl. Sports Sci. Res. 5:100–107, 1992.

training and competition will be limited only if there is evidence that performance is compromised to an extent that may lead to injury or that health is seriously threatened.

6. If the athlete admits that a problem exists, referral to a health professional (who is experienced with eating disorders in athletes) is essential for treatment.

7. If the coach or trainer strongly suspects that an eating problem exists and the athlete denies it, a mandatory meeting with a health professional for further evaluation is necessary. Explain to the athlete that pursuing help may be the single most important factor to achieve or preserve success in his or her sport.

8. Recognize that eating disorders are complex and treatment is a lengthy process. Show athletes that you understand that their eating problems do not represent failure or a lack of effort.

There are several strategies that are important to **avoid** when approaching an athlete with an eating problem:

1. Never ignore the problem, hoping it will disappear with time. The problem will not correct itself and only becomes more serious and difficult to treat.

2. Never initiate a discussion with an athlete's teammates about the problem. If you are approached by athletes, thank them for their concern and reassure them that you will speak with the athlete privately.

3. The coach should never punish athletes by dismissing them from the team or otherwise reprimanding them for an eating disorder. This will only make their eating problem worse.

4. Do not be reluctant to seek outside assistance from health professionals. Discussing the athlete's problem in confidence with a professional may be reassuring and will help you to determine treatment alternatives. Another possibility is to have a health professional give an informal talk about eating

disorders to the team to discuss eating and weight-related concerns. Educational materials can be handed out that highlight the symptoms and consequences of eating disorders and where athletes can go to get help.

5. Never abandon the athlete after he or she agrees to seek treatment. Performance will most likely decrease during treatment, and expectations should be adjusted accordingly. This will minimize the anxiety the athlete already feels and will aid recovery.

COMPLICATIONS OF EATING DISORDERS

Eating disorders are a serious medical problem. The physiological and psychological consequences of eating disorders are considerable and can include death. Most complications of anorexia nervosa occur as a direct or indirect result of starvation and include malnutrition, anemia, decreased heart mass, heart rhythm disturbances due to electrolyte imbalances, and even death. Most complications of bulimia nervosa occur due to bingeing and purging and include erosion of tooth enamel, tears in the esophagus, aspiration pneumonia, and heart failure. Tables 14-2 and 14-3 highlight key medical complications of anorexia nervosa and bulimia nervosa.

In the early 1990s, a strong relationship was recognized between eating disorders, amenorrhea (menstruation stops), and osteoporosis. This has been termed the Female Athlete Triad. The Triad occurs in physically active girls and women as well as elite athletes. The components of the Triad are interrelated in cause, progression, and outcome. Alone or in combination, Triad disorders can reduce physical performance and have serious medical and psychological consequences.

All other causes of amenorrhea must be excluded by a physician. Reduced training, increased calorie intake, weight gain, calcium supplementation (1,500 milligrams of elemental calcium),

---

TABLE 14-2
Health Consequences of Anorexia Nervosa

- Malnutrition and slowed metabolism.
- Abnormally slow heart rate and low blood pressure. The risk for heart failure increases as heart rate and blood prssure levels decrease.
- Loss of body fat and muscle.
- Intolerance to cold.
- Dehydration which can result in kidney failure.
- Fatigue, overall weakness, fainting spells.
- Abdominal pain, slow stomach emptying.
- Hair loss; dry hair and skin.
- Growth of a fine layer of hair on the body in an effort to keep the body warm.
- Menstruation becomes irregular or stops completely.
- Loss of bone density that may lead to dry, brittle bones that are susceptible to fracture.

---

and hormone replacement therapy may be recommended to help restore menses and protect bone. However, bone mineral density may not return to normal levels. Poor nutrition and amenorrhea may reduce skeletal accretion during the critical years of bone formation in the adolescent athlete, placing the athlete at risk for stress fractures and premature osteoporosis.

PREVENTION OF EATING DISORDERS

Society as a whole needs to be educated about healthy weight and realistic body image. Young women, in particular, should be encouraged to develop a sense of self-esteem and self-worth that is not based on their body shape and size. This will help them to resist the pressure to conform to unrealistic and unattainable standards of appearance.

Women (and men) who have been repeatedly unsuccessful at weight-loss attempts may want to consider abandoning weight

---

TABLE 14-3
Health Consequences of Bulimia Nervosa

Complications due to vomiting:

- Malnutrition and changes in metabolism.
- Dehydration.
- Electrolyte imbalances of sodium and potassium that can lead to irregular heartbeats and possibly heart failure and death.
- Tooth decay by stomach acids.
- Salivary gland enlargement.
- Inflammation, tears, of the esophagus or stomach.
- Peptic ulcers and inflammation of the pancreas.

Complications due to diuretics abuse:

- Electrolyte imbalances of sodium and potassium that can lead to irregular heartbeats and possibly heart failure and death.
- Dehydration.
- Fatigue.
- Muscle weakness.

Complications due to laxative abuse:

- Dependence on laxatives.
- Diarrhea, constipation.
- Abdominal pain: bloating, gas, cramping.
- Irregular bowel movements and constipation.

---

loss as a goal altogether. Instead of dieting, they can focus on normalizing their eating behaviors, eating more healthfully, becoming more physically active, and building positive self-esteem.

Since there are many contributing factors to eating disorders (the exact cause is unknown), it is a challenge to determine preventive strategies. It seems that education is key to heightened awareness and understanding that will facilitate early detection and treatment of eating disorders. Although there have been some notable cases when athletes have performed successfully despite eating problems, these are short-lived or exceptions. Athletes need to know that an eating disorder is a threat to health as well as performance.

Coaches, parents, friends, and teammates need to recognize the role that they may play in contributing to an eating disorder. Inappropriate remarks about an athlete's body size or need for weight loss (without offering guidance from a professional on how to do this healthfully) can strongly influence his or her eating behaviors and may trigger the development of a serious problem.

In an effort to achieve or maintain a reasonable competitive weight, athletes need nutritional counseling by a qualified sports nutritionist. The sports nutritionist can then individualize the weight-control program and provide sport-specific nutritional guidance. Nutrition education programs for athletic groups should include candid discussions of the health and performance consequences of eating disorders. Educational materials should include the signs and complications of eating disorders and where the athlete can get help.

Finally, the sports community must consider the demand placed on female athletes to achieve unrealistic weights and body shapes. When one considers the medical complications of anorexia and bulimia, the emotional distress suffered by the athlete, the negative impact on those close to the athlete, and the extraordinary costs of treatment, eating disorders are one of the most serious problems facing female athletes. Where does the responsibility lie? With coaches? sports judges? parents? the media? athletes? All may play a significant role in placing a premium on thinness.

15

NUTRITION FOR
THE YOUNG
ATHLETE

W
hether it's training for an upcoming soccer game, or play-
ing a backyard game of catch, children's athletic performance, development, and growth depend on eating the
right foods. Children are not miniature adults—parents and
coaches need to consider the special needs of young athletes for
training and performance. Table 15-1 provides the Young Athlete's Bill of Rights. Read on to learn the basics for keeping active
children fueled and hydrated for peak performance and fun.

PHYSICAL GROWTH

All children should have their height and weight plotted by a
health professional on the National Center for Health Statistics
(NCHS) growth charts. These charts are routinely used by pedia-
tricians to evaluate growth of children and adolescents. Increases
in height and weight during the early school-age years are small
compared with the rapid growth observed during infancy and
adolescence. Young children typically grow 2 to 3 inches and gain
3 to 6 pounds each year. At puberty, however, children undergo
hormonal changes that mark the beginning of adolescence. These

TABLE 15-1
Young Athlete's Bill of Rights

1. The right to have the opportunity to participate in sports regardless of ability level.
2. The right to participate at a level commensurate with the child's developmental level.
3. The right to have qualified adult leadership.
4. The right to participate in a safe and healthy environment.
5. The right of each child to share leadership and decision making.
6. The right to play as a child and not as an adult.
7. The right to proper preparation for participation in sports.
8. The right to equal opportunity to strive for success.
9. The right to be treated with dignity by all involved.
10. The right to have fun through sports.

Source: "So What's Good About Sports?" *Am J Dis Child* 1988; 142:143.
© 1988 AMA. Reprinted with permission from the American Medical Association.

hormonal changes cause them to grow rapidly. It is especially important to make certain that children entering puberty are meeting their nutritional needs.

Tanner Stages of Development

The rate and age of sexual maturation is highly variable and differs within and between the sexes. To help monitor maturing children, the Tanner stages of sexual development (sexual maturity ratings) can be used (Table 15-2). This numerical system has been established for describing children in terms of how their bodies are changing and developing sexually.

Although formal Tanner staging is determined by a physician, other characteristics can be used to estimate the level of sexual maturity. For girls, the rapid period of growth is completed when menstruation begins at Tanner stage 4. Boys grow fastest between Tanner stages 3 and 4. Following the growth spurt in stage 4, the boy has enough circulating hormones in the

TABLE 15-2
Tanner Stages of Development

STAGE		BOYS	GIRLS
1		Prepubescent	Prepubescent
2		First appearance of pubic hair	First appearance of pubic hair
	Peak Growth Spurt in Girls	Growth of genitalia	Development of genitalia
		Increased activity of sweat glands	Increased activity of sweat glands
3		Pubic hair extends to scrotum	Pubic hair thicker, coarser, curly
		Growth and pigmentation of genitalia	Breasts enlarge and pigmentation continues
	Peak Growth Spurt in Boys	Changes in voice Beginning of acne	Genitalia well developed Beginning of acne
4		Pubic hair thickens, facial hair begins	Pubic hair abundant, armpit hair begins
		Growth and pigmentation of genitalia	Breasts enlarge and mature
		Voice deepens	Genitalia assume adult structure
		Acne may be severe	Acne may be severe Menarche begins
5		Increased distribution of hair	Increased pubic hair distribution
		Genitalia fully mature	Breasts fully mature
		Acne may persist and increase	Increased severity of acne (if present)

blood to facilitate muscle mass and show signs of facial hair. Upon examination, if a boy has only "peach fuzz" for facial hair and/or has not started shaving, he probably has not completed his growth spurt.

EATING BEHAVIORS AND PATTERNS

When children reach elementary school, they develop eating patterns that are more independent of the influence and scrutiny of their parents. New activities and friends begin to influence choices as children are exposed to a variety of new foods and different social situations. School-age children tend to be repetitious in their food choices, so the food groups they include in their diets remain relatively constant from month to month.

Many school-age children skip breakfast. Usually, the main reason is lack of time. However, children who eat breakfast have a better attitude, school record, and problem-solving ability compared to children who do not eat breakfast. In addition, breakfast helps to replenish liver glycogen stores depleted during an overnight fast. This ensures that the child has adequate energy stores for afternoon training. Children should be encouraged to find foods they like for breakfast. These do not need to be traditional foods. Food composition, not social tradition, is the best strategy.

Some athletes such as figure skaters practice early in the morning before they go to school. Under these circumstances, the child should be encouraged to have a small snack before activity such as fruit juice and toast, oatmeal and fruit, or bagel with peanut butter and jelly followed by additional carbohydrate-rich and fluids after activity.

The child's lunch may be provided by the school or brought from home. The federal government requires its school lunch program to provide approximately one-third of the recommended dietary allowances for children. Many changes have been implemented in the school lunch program in recent years. For example, popular items such as pizza, tacos, macaroni and cheese, and hamburgers are often included on the menu, fresh fruits are provided as an alternative to desserts like cake and cookies, and skim milk is offered in addition to whole milk.

School lunch may be more nutritious than a lunch brought from home. This is because box lunches typically contain less variety and include only favorite foods. In addition, they are limited to foods that travel well and do not require heating or refrigeration. Even when a nutritious lunch is packed at home, the parent does not necessarily know what portion is eaten, traded, or thrown away.

Food choices are typically influenced by the child's friends. To gain a better understanding of what the child eats, parents should ask children if they eat lunch with their friends and why they prefer certain foods.

Snacks may contribute significantly to the child's nutrient intake and eating style. The quality of snacks eaten may determine whether nutrient requirements are being met. Therefore, the frequency of snacking and type of snacks are important considerations. For example, does the child snack during the morning and/or before going to bed? What are her or his favorite snacks? Are they prepared at home or purchased from a vending machine?

For most athletes, practice is held after school. After a training session, many children come home from school exhausted and hungry. Bakery products, soft drinks, candy, and chips often top their list of favorites and are the most frequently chosen snack foods. It is important that nutritious foods, especially those that are quick and easy to prepare, are available at typical snack times. In addition, the child should be encouraged to rehydrate by consuming water and fruit juices.

DIETARY RECOMMENDATIONS FOR YOUNG ATHLETES

What is the most appropriate diet for the young athlete? Adequate energy and nutrients should be obtained from a diet that emphasizes nutrient-dense carbohydrates and moderate amounts of protein and fat to support growth and physical activity. This can be achieved by planning intake to include a variety of foods from each of the major food groups as illustrated by the Food Guide Pyramid. The key messages of variety, balance, and moderation in food choices should be promoted. Especially for the child, the pyramid serves as a visual guide for choosing foods and helping to plan healthful meals.

Each day, the young athlete should consume at least 2 to 3 servings from the milk group, 2 to 3 servings from the meat/protein group, 4 servings from the vegetable group, 3 servings from the fruit group, and 9 servings from the bread/grain group. Foods at the top of the Pyramid that contain the majority of their calories from fat or sugars may be consumed occasionally in addition to, not in place of, other nutrient dense foods.

In general, providing servings within these recommended ranges will supply the necessary calories (2,200 calories) and nutrients that most active children require. However, depending on the frequency, intensity, and duration of physical activity, the exercising child may need an additional 500 to 1,000 calories each day. Children should be encouraged to distribute calories throughout the day at regular mealtimes and snacks. This will ensure the presence of readily available sources of energy to support training activity.

How Parents Can Help Their Children Eat Better

Young children rely for the most part on the foods that are brought into the house. In addition to having the parent purchase more healthful foods, favorite foods can be made more nutritionally dense or acceptable substitutions can be made with similar foods. There are many different food choices available that will supply adequate amounts of vitamins and minerals for even the fussiest of eaters. To increase nutrient density, encourage small, gradual changes that are acceptable to the child. For example, fortified cereals can be served rather than sugary ones, oatmeal raisin cookies can be offered instead of chocolate cream cookies, fruit-flavored frozen yogurt can be served for dessert as an alternative to ice cream. Parents can pack snacks and fluids for before and after practice so that the child does not have to rely on vending machines.

Parents can explain basic facts about the different food groups and how the foods relate to exercise. Attempts to teach children nutrition concepts and information should take into account their developmental level. For example, parents can explain that carbohydrate foods like bread and pasta provide energy for the muscles and that dairy foods like milk help build strong bones. The objective is to increase the child's awareness, not enforce stringent guidelines.

Variety and balance in the family menu will underscore the importance of eating different foods to provide the range of nutrients necessary for growth and development. Ideally, this is achieved by regularly scheduled meals at home plus nutritious snacks. However, preparing routine meals and snacks may not always be possible. An important issue facing parents with children in sports is how to provide nutritious meals around hectic practice schedules. Workouts may interfere with home meals, resulting in a greater reliance on convenient fast foods or the child eating alone after the family has finished. Children need guidance on how to make nutritious choices at fast-food restaurants.

SPECIAL FLUID NEEDS OF CHILDREN

Children and adults react to heat and exercise differently. Since children are smaller than adults, they don't sweat as much and are less able to cool their bodies adequately. Also, children absorb heat from their surroundings more easily than do adults. Acclimatization to exercise in the heat is more gradual in children compared to adolescents or adults.

All of these factors increase the risk of dehydration in children. Therefore, fluids play a critical role in maintaining health and performance of the child athlete. Heatstroke ranks second among reported causes of death in high school athletes. By educating young athletes about the importance of fluids and how to keep hydrated, heatstroke can be prevented.

If a child tires easily and repeatedly in practice and appears irritable, and performance suddenly declines, dehydration and/or inadequate calorie intake may be the cause. The following are signs of dehydration: dry lips and tongue, sunken eyes, bright colored or dark urine, infrequent urination, and apathy or lack of energy.

Fluid Guidelines for Exercising Children

To prevent dehydration, encourage children to drink cool fluids before, during, and after physical activity. See Figure 15-1 for specific guidelines.

- Encourage children to drink on a schedule—at least 4 ounces every 15 to 20 minutes. Thirst is not an accurate measure of the body's need for fluid—when children are thirsty, they are already dehydrated. Giving children personalized squeeze bottles promotes fluid intake.
- Supervision of fluid intake is essential for children because they do not instinctively drink enough fluid to replace water losses. During prolonged exercise, children and adolescents may not recognize the symptoms of heat strain and push themselves to the point of heat-related illness.
- Children should be weighed before and after exercise. Make sure that they drink 16 to 24 ounces of fluid for every pound of weight lost.
- Although plain water is inexpensive and readily available, children are more likely to drink sufficient amounts if they are given flavored fluids such as sports drinks. A sports drink such as Gatorade supplies energy and encourages drinking by "turning on" thirst.
- Avoid beverages that are higher in sugar, such as fruit juices and soft drinks. They are absorbed slower and increase the chance of stomach cramps, nausea, and diarrhea.

FIGURE 15-1
Fluid Guidelines for Young Athletes

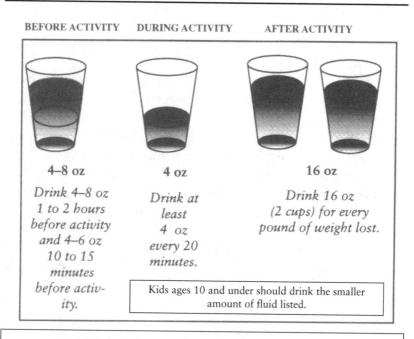

BEFORE ACTIVITY	DURING ACTIVITY	AFTER ACTIVITY
4–8 oz	4 oz	16 oz
Drink 4–8 oz 1 to 2 hours before activity and 4–6 oz 10 to 15 minutes before activity.	*Drink at least 4 oz every 20 minutes.*	*Drink 16 oz (2 cups) for every pound of weight lost.*

Kids ages 10 and under should drink the smaller amount of fluid listed.

Source: Adapted from F. Meyer and O. Bar-Or, *Sports Med.* 18 (1): 4–9, 1994.

Preventing Heat Disorders in Children

In addition to ensuring that the young athlete drinks enough fluids, adults can take a number of precautions to significantly reduce the risk of heat injury in children:

- Adjust the timing of practice depending on the weather. Schedule workouts for the coolest time of the day (before 10 A.M., after 6 P.M.) especially in warm, humid conditions. Extreme heat and humidity are valid reasons to cancel practice or competition.

- Allow athletes to gradually adjust to harder workouts and warmer weather.
- When possible, avoid excessive clothing, taping, or padding on hot/humid days. On such days, schedule football workouts with padding and other gear for early morning instead of afternoon.
- Schedule frequent fluid and rest breaks in the shade. Insist that all athletes drink a certain amount of fluid before returning to practice.
- Never withhold fluid as a disciplinary measure. Fluid should be available at all times of training and competition.
- Because volume of sweat loss varies, weigh athletes before and after exercise to estimate total water loss during practice.
- Be aware of children and adolescents who may be at increased risk for heat disorders due to obesity, poor conditioning, or other chronic health problems.
- Discourage using dehydration practices to lose weight and encourage proper hydration.

WEIGHT-CONTROL PRACTICES

In pursuit of athletic prowess, healthy nutritional practices may be disregarded by parents and coaches who are not well informed about a child's stage of maturation, nutritional needs, emotions, and physical ability.

Unfortunately, some parents and coaches have misconceptions about how much and what types of foods young children should eat. Some encourage their children to eat excessively, with the erroneous belief that this will build strength and endurance more quickly. To the contrary, indiscriminate consumption, in which food intake exceeds the child's calorie requirement, may be the start of a lifelong struggle with being overweight.

At the other extreme are parents who adopt a restrictive diet that may endanger the health of the child. Given the current recommendations to reduce fat intake, many parents may encourage their children to do the same in an attempt to minimize the risk of heart disease. However, the American College of Pediatrics Committee on Nutrition does not recommend low-fat diets for young children. Rather, it recommends that children receive 30% of total calories from fat. Restriction of intake to lower levels will hinder adequate growth and development.

Diets restricted in fat and cholesterol reduce the intake of red meat and milk, both of which are major sources of protein, iron, calcium, and other minerals necessary for growth. Parents can encourage long-term healthful habits without compromising growth needs by offering foods with moderate amounts of unsaturated fats versus foods high in saturated fat.

For some sports, weight-related demands placed on athletic children by a parent or coach can be misguided and extreme. Children may be told to sweat off extra pounds by fluid restriction and exercising in a hot environment or encouraged to chronically restrict food intake in an effort to promote weight loss. Instead of improved performance, the result can be fatigue, heat exhaustion, and health problems. Nutritional needs for growth and development must be placed before athletic considerations.

WORKING WITH THE OBESE YOUNG ATHLETE

Obesity (a weight that is 20% above healthy body weight) is an increasing problem among children and adolescents in the United States and occurs as a result of a complex interaction of genetic and environmental factors. Children are also becoming obese at younger ages, and obesity that occurs earlier and persists throughout childhood is more difficult to treat. Even though complications related to obesity are considerably less for children and adolescents than for adults, obesity that continues into adulthood may lead to chronic diseases such as hypertension, diabetes, and heart disease. From a psychological standpoint, a major concern accompanying chronic childhood obesity is the potential for emotional upset and loss of self-esteem caused by the stigma of being overweight.

Although obesity is an important health problem and prevalence is increasing, efforts by coaches or parents to eliminate excess body fat by requiring the obese child to exercise excessively can be too sudden or too extreme. The obese child participating in sports needs a medically supervised weight-control program that focuses on weight monitoring, calorie reduction, and gradual increased activity. Several strategies for working with the obese child during a weight-reduction plan are outlined below for coaches and parents.

Coaches

- Never single out obese children by asking them to run extra laps or exercise longer than other children.
- Never restrict fluids for any child.
- Never refer to the child as being obese or chubby, especially in front of his or her teammates.
- Watch for signs of heat distress. Obese children are at a higher risk for heat disorders than normal-weight children.
- Be patient with regard to weight- and physical-activity-related expectations.
- Encourage children to feel good about themselves—regardless of talent, body size, or shape.

Parents

- Work with a health professional who has experience with weight control and young athletes to develop a plan for your child that is medically sound and nutritionally balanced.
- Encourage and support recommendations made by the health professional.
- Do not single out the obese child in the family by serving special foods or imposing restrictions. Include the whole family in making healthier, low-fat choices.

- Make mealtime pleasant. Encourage the child to eat slowly and to enjoy whatever she or he eats.
- Never give foods as a reward or withhold them as a punishment.
- Do not tell a child he or she is "on a diet" and that certain foods are "good" and others are "bad."
- Involve the child in shopping and food preparation.
- Never discuss the child's weight in front of others.
- Ask the advice of a health professional on the issue of other siblings or friends teasing the obese child.
- For the entire family, discourage eating meals and snacks while watching television.
- Examine your own dietary intake and attitudes toward food. Take an active role in establishing a healthy outlook toward exercise, eating, and body image with your child.

DIETARY SUPPLEMENTS

Parents can help children choose diets that meet their vitamin and mineral needs by utilizing the Food Guide Pyramid. Dietary supplements (vitamin/mineral supplements, ergogenic aids, and herbs) are not recommended for children, as the full short- and long-term impact of these substances on young, growing bodies is virtually unknown. Keep in mind that dietary supplements are not regulated for safety, effectiveness, potency, or purity.

Unfortunately, many well-meaning but misinformed parents and coaches advise children to take supplements in an effort to promote early athletic development, improve performance, and provide "nutrition insurance." However, eventual maturity and athletic ability do not depend on how early the child begins adolescence. Also, dietary supplements don't "speed up" a child's growth and development.

Large doses of vitamins and minerals can be dangerous, and growing individuals are at greater risk of experiencing adverse effects. Providing children with vitamin/mineral supplements can also encourage faulty eating habits. Young athletes may assume that their morning dose of supplements provides them with all the nutrients they need so that they can eat candy and soda instead of cereal and milk.

Another disadvantage of supplement use is that young athletes may erroneously associate improvements in performance with whatever supplements they may happen to be taking. They may be less likely to attribute their progress to training, hard work, and a balanced diet. Supplements also don't give athletes a competitive advantage or make up for a lack of training or talent.

To move away from this reliance on "supplement insurance," young athletes need to feel confident about eating "ordinary foods." Parents, coaches, and health professionals must emphasize how regular foods promote muscle growth and optimal performance. From a practical standpoint, this is an important reason to encourage young athletes to keep records of what they eat, how they train, and how their performance improves. These records can be used to illustrate the importance of good dietary and training habits as the cause of improvement, rather than leaving the child to erroneously associate athletic accomplishments with a pill.

For the young athlete, as for all athletes, the key to health and performance cannot be found in any one food or supplement. Instead, the child should be encouraged to consume a wide variety of foods from the Food Guide Pyramid to obtain the many different nutrients the body requires for optimal growth and development.

Appendix A

FAST-FOOD CHOICES FOR BREAKFAST, LUNCH, AND DINNER

The following two tables, A-1 and A-2, list lower-fat, high-carbohydrate breakfast, lunch, and dinner choices at selected fast-food restaurants.

TABLE A-1
High-Carbohydrate Breakfast Food Choices
at Selected Fast-Food Restaurants

FOOD ITEM	SERVING SIZE	KCAL	CARBO-HYDRATE	PROTEIN	FAT	EXCHANGES
CARL'S JR.						
English muffin with margarine	2 oz.	190	63%	13%	24%	2 starch, 1 fat
Bran/blueberry muffin	4.8–4.2 oz.	310–340	67–72%	13–14%	20–24%	3½ starch, 1 fat
Orange juice	9 oz.	90	93%	7%	0%	1½ fruit
McDONALD'S						
Egg McMuffin	4.8 oz.	280	40%	25%	35%	2 starch, 2 medium fat meat
Cheerios	¾ cup	80	70%	15%	15%	1 starch
Wheaties	¾ cup	90	84%	9%	7%	1 starch
Fat-free apple bran muffin	2.6 oz.	180	89%	11%	0%	2½ starch
Hot cakes Syrup	1 order 1½ fl. oz.	250 120	80%	13%	7%	3 starch, ½ fat 2 fruit
Apple, grapefruit, orange juice	6 oz.	80	95%	5%	0%	1 fruit
ARBY'S						
Cinnamon nut danish	3.5 oz.	360	67%	6%	27%	4 starch, 2 fat
Blueberry muffin	2.7 oz.	240	67%	7%	26%	2½ starch, 1 fat

TABLE A-2
Lower-Fat, or High-Carbohydrate Lunch and Dinner Food Choices at Selected Fast-Food Restaurants

FOOD ITEM	SERVING SIZE	KCAL	CARBO- HYDRATE	PROTEIN	FAT	EXCHANGES
ARBY'S						
French dip sandwich	5.4 oz.	368	38%	25%	37%	2 starch, 2 medium fat meat, 1 fat
Grilled chicken barbecue sandwich	7.1 oz.	386	49%	21%	30%	3 starch, 3 medium fat meat
Hot ham and cheese sandwich	6 oz.	355	39%	26%	35%	2 starch, 3 medium fat meat
Light roast chicken deluxe sandwich	6.8 oz.	276	48%	46%	6%	2 starch, 2½ lean meat
Light roast turkey deluxe sandwich	6.8 oz.	260	51%	42%	7%	2 starch, 2 lean meat
Roast chicken salad	14 oz.	204	47%	22%	31%	1 starch, 2 vegetable, 1 medium fat meat
Light Italian dressing	2 oz.	23	52%	0%	38%	½ fat
Baked potato	8.5 oz.	240	83%	10%	7%	3 starch
Garden salad	11.6 oz.	117	38%	24%	38%	2 vegetable, 1 fat
Lumberjack mixed vegetable soup	8 oz.	89	58%	12%	30%	1 starch
Old-fashioned chicken soup	8 oz.	99	61%	21%	18%	1 starch

(continued on next page)

TABLE A-2 (continued)
Lower-Fat, or High-Carbohydrate Lunch and Dinner Food Choices at Selected Fast-Food Restaurants

FOOD ITEM	SERVING SIZE	KCAL	CARBO-HYDRATE	PROTEIN	FAT	EXCHANGES
BURGER KING						
Hamburger	3.6 oz.	260	43%	22%	35%	2 starch, 2 medium fat meat
BK Broiler chicken sandwich	5.4 oz.	280	41%	27%	32%	2 starch, 2 medium fat meat
Chicken salad without dressing	9 oz.	142	23%	52%	25%	1 vegetable, 2 lean meat
Light Italian dressing	2 oz.	30	80%	0%	20%	½ fat
Lemon pie	3.2 oz.	290	68%	7%	25%	3 starch, 1 fat
CARL'S JR.						
Hamburger	4.3 oz.	320	41%	18%	39%	2 starch, 2 medium fat meat
Charbroiler BBQ chicken sandwich	11 oz.	310	44%	39%	17%	2 starch, 3 lean meat
Teriyaki chicken sandwich	8.3 oz.	330	51%	33%	16%	1½ starch, 2½ lean meat
Santa Fe chicken sandwich	7.8 oz.	540	57%	22%	22%	5 starch, 2½ lean meat
Lite potato	10 oz.	290	83%	14%	3%	4 starch
Garden salad to go	4.8 oz.	50	32%	14%	54%	1 vegetable

TABLE A-2 (continued)
Lower-Fat, or High-Carbohydrate Lunch and Dinner Food Choices at Selected Fast-Food Restaurants

FOOD ITEM	SERVING SIZE	KCAL	CARBO-HYDRATE	PROTEIN	FAT	EXCHANGES
CARL'S JR. (continued)						
Chicken salad to go	12 oz.	200	16%	48%	36%	1 vegetable, 3 lean meat
Reduced-calorie French dressing	1 oz.	40	55%	0%	45%	1 fat
Salsa	1 oz.	8	100%	—	—	—
KENTUCKY FRIED CHICKEN						

Side items that are low in fat and high in carbohydrate:

FOOD ITEM	SERVING SIZE	KCAL	CARBO-HYDRATE	PROTEIN	FAT	EXCHANGES
Corn on cob	2.6 oz.	90	71%	8%	20%	1 starch
Baked beans	3 oz.	105	69%	23%	8%	1 starch
Mashed potatoes with gravy	3.5 oz.	71	68%	7%	25%	1 starch

Note: Despite different coatings, all KFC chicken is fried. Therefore, calories from fat range between 48% and 59% (even skin-free crispy).

FOOD ITEM	SERVING SIZE	KCAL	CARBO-HYDRATE	PROTEIN	FAT	EXCHANGES
McDONALD'S						
Hamburger	3.6 oz.	255	47%	21%	32%	2 starch, 1 medium fat meat, 1 fat
McLean Deluxe	7.7 oz	320	44%	28%	28%	2 starch, 3 lean meat
Chicken fajitas	2.9 oz.	190	42%	20%	38%	1 starch, 1 lean meat, 1 fat
Cheese pizza	2.6 oz. (1 slice)	178	54%	11%	35%	1½ starch, 1 medium fat meat

(continued on next page)

TABLE A-2 (continued)
Lower-Fat, or High-Carbohydrate Lunch and Dinner Food Choices at Selected Fast-Food Restaurants

FOOD ITEM	SERVING SIZE	KCAL	CARBO-HYDRATE	PROTEIN	FAT	EXCHANGES
McDONALD'S (continued)						
Chunky chicken salad	9 oz.	150	19%	57%	24%	1 vegetable, 3 lean meat
Garden salad	6.6 oz.	50	48%	16%	36%	1 vegetable
Lite vinaigrette	2 oz.	48	67%	0%	33%	1 fat
DOMINO'S PIZZA						
Cheese pizza	2 slices of a large (5.5 oz.)	376	60%	16%	24%	4 starch, 2 medium fat meat
Vegetable pizza	2 slices of a large (5.5 oz.)	498	48%	18%	34%	4 starch, 3 medium fat meat, 1 fat
Ham pizza	2 slices of medium pizza (5.5 oz.)	417	55%	22%	23%	4 starch, 2 medium fat meat
PIZZA HUT PIZZA						
Thin crispy* Veggie Lover's pizza	2 slices of medium pizza	384	42%	20%	38%	2 starch, 3 medium fat meat
Cheese pizza	2 slices of medium pizza	446	34%	26%	40%	2 starch, 3 medium fat meat, 2 fat

* Hand-tossed pizza has similar values; pan pizza is significantly higher in calories.

TACO BELL						
Bean burrito	6.7 oz.	359	60%	12%	28%	3½ starch, 1 medium fat meat, 1 fat

TABLE A-2 (continued)
Lower-Fat, or High-Carbohydrate Lunch and Dinner Food Choices at Selected Fast-Food Restaurants

FOOD ITEM	SERVING SIZE	KCAL	CARBO-HYDRATE	PROTEIN	FAT	EXCHANGES
TACO BELL (continued)						
Chicken burrito	6 oz.	334	46%	22%	32%	2½ starch, 2 medium fat meat
Border lights*	(have 50% less fat than comparable products)					
Light taco salad with chips	21 oz.	680	48%	19%	33%	5 starch, 3½ lean meat
Light soft taco	3.25 oz.	180	42%	33%	25%	1 starch, 1½ lean meat

* Available at selected locations

FOOD ITEM	SERVING SIZE	KCAL	CARBO-HYDRATE	PROTEIN	FAT	EXCHANGES
WENDY'S						
Grilled hamburger	4 oz.	270	50%	20%	30%	2 starch, 1½ medium fat meat
Grilled chicken sandwich	6.25 oz.	290	48%	30%	22%	2 starch, 1 vegetable, 2 lean meat
Baked potato	10 oz.	300	92%	7%	0%	4 starch
Chili	8 oz. (small)	190	44%	28%	28%	1½ starch, 2 lean meat
Grilled chicken salad	12 oz.	200	18%	46%	36%	2 vegetable, 3 lean meat

At the salad bar, avoid higher-fat items such as bacon bits, cheese, coleslaw, chicken, seafood, tuna salad (with oil or mayonnaise), potato or pasta salad (withoil or mayonnaise), pepperoni, luncheon meats, diced, and nuts.

(continued on next page)

TABLE A-2 (continued)
Lower-Fat, or High-Carbohydrate Lunch and Dinner Food Choices at Selected Fast-Food Restaurants

FOOD ITEM	SERVING SIZE	KCAL	CARBO-HYDRATE	PROTEIN	FAT	EXCHANGES
SUBWAY						
COLD SUBS, 6-inch						
Veggie Delite	182 gm.	237	44 gm.	9 gm.	3 gm.	3 starch
Turkey	239 gm.	289	46 gm.	18 gm.	4 gm.	3 starch, 2 very lean meat
Subway Club	253 gm.	312	46 gm.	21 gm.	5 gm.	2 starch, 2 very lean meat
Roast beef	239 gm.	303	45 gm.	20 gm.	5 gm.	3 starch, 2 very lean meat
Turkey breast & ham	239 gm.	295	46 gm.	18 gm.	5 gm.	3 starch, 2 very lean meat
Ham	239 gm.	302	45 gm.	19 gm.	5 gm.	3 starch, 2 very lean meat
Seafood & crab	253 gm.	347	45 gm.	20 gm.	10 gm.	3 starch, 2 lean meat
HOT SUBS, 6-inch						
Roasted chicken breast	253 gm.	348	47 gm.	27 gm.	6 gm.	3 starch, 3 very lean meat
Subway Melt	258 gm.	382	46 gm.	23 gm.	12 gm.	3 starch, 2 medium fat meat
Meat ball	287 gm.	419	51 gm.	19 gm.	16 gm.	3½ starch, 2 medium fat meat
Steak & cheese	264 gm.	398	47 gm.	30 gm.	10 gm.	3 starch, 2 lean meat
SALADS						
Veggie Delite	260 gm.	51	10 gm.	2 gm.	0	½ starch or 2 vegetables

TABLE A-2 (continued)
Lower-Fat, or High-Carbohydrate Lunch and Dinner Food Choices at Selected Fast-Food Restaurants

FOOD ITEM	SERVING SIZE	KCAL	CARBO-HYDRATE	PROTEIN	FAT	EXCHANGES
SUBWAY (continued)						
SALADS (continued)						
Turkey breast	316 gm.	102	12 gm.	11 gm.	2 gm.	2 vegetable, 1 lean meat
Ham	316 gm.	116	11 gm.	12 gm.	3 gm.	2 vegetable, 1 lean meat
OPTIONAL FIXINGS						
Light mayonnaise	1 tsp.	18	0	0	2 gm.	—
Mustard	2 tsp.	8	1 gm.	1 gm.	0	—
Vinegar	1 tsp.	1	0	0	00	—

Appendix B

CALORIC EXPENDITURES

The following table lists approximate caloric expenditures per minute for various physical activities.

APPENDIX B: APPROXIMATE CALORIC EXPENDITURE PER MINUTE FOR VARIOUS PHYSICAL ACTIVITIES*

| Body Weight in kilograms | 45 | 50 | 55 | 59 | 64 | 68 | 73 | 77 | 82 | 86 | 91 | 95 | 100 |
Body Weight in pounds	100	110	120	130	140	150	160	170	180	190	200	210	220
SEDENTARY ACTIVITIES													
Lying quietly	.99	1.1	1.2	1.3	1.4	1.5	1.6	1.7	1.8	1.9	2.0	2.1	2.2
Sitting and writing	1.2	1.4	1.5	1.7	1.8	1.9	2.0	2.2	2.3	2.4	2.5	2.7	2.8
Standing with light work	2.7	3.0	3.3	3.5	3.8	4.1	4.4	4.6	4.9	5.2	5.4	5.7	6.0
PHYSICAL ACTIVITIES													
Archery	3.1	3.5	3.8	4.1	4.5	4.8	5.1	5.4	5.7	6.0	6.4	6.7	7.0
Badminton													
Recreational singles	3.6	4.0	4.4	4.7	5.1	5.4	5.8	6.2	6.6	6.9	7.3	7.6	8.0
Competitive	5.9	6.4	7.0	7.6	8.2	8.8	9.4	10.0	10.l6	11.2	11.8	12.4	13.0
Baseball													
Player	3.1	3.4	3.8	4.1	4.4	4.7	5.0	5.3	5.6	5.9	6.3	6.6	6.9
Pitcher	3.9	4.3	4.7	5.1	5.5	5.9	6.3	6.7	7.1	7.4	7.9	8.2	8.6
Basketball													
Recreational	4.9	5.5	6.0	6.5	7.0	7.5	8.0	8.5	9.0	9.5	10.0	10.5	11.0
Vigorous competition	6.5	7.2	7.8	8.5	9.2	9.9	10.5	11.2	11.9	12.5	13.2	13.8	14.5
Bicycling, level													
(mph) (min/mile)													
5 12:00	1.9	2.1	2.3	2.5	2.7	2.9	3.1	3.3	3.5	3.7	3.9	4.1	4.3
10 6:00	4.2	4.6	5.1	5.5	5.9	6.4	6.8	7.2	7.6	8.1	8.5	8.9	9.4
15 4:00	7.3	8.0	8.7	9.5	10.0	10.9	11.6	12.4	13.1	13.8	14.5	15.3	16.0
20 3:00	10.7	11.7	12.8	13.9	14.9	16.0	17.1	18.1	19.2	20.3	21.3	22.4	23.5

Adapted from Williams, M. H. *Nutrition for Fitness and Sport*, 3rd ed. Wm. C. Brown Publishers, 1992.

APPENDIX B: APPROXIMATE CALORIC EXPENDITURE PER MINUTE FOR VARIOUS PHYSICAL ACTIVITIES*

| Body Weight in kilograms | 45 | 50 | 55 | 59 | 64 | 68 | 73 | 77 | 82 | 86 | 91 | 95 | 100 |
Body Weight in pounds	100	110	120	130	140	150	160	170	180	190	200	210	220
PHYSICAL ACTIVITIES													
Canoeing													
(mph) (min/mile)													
2.5 24	1.9	2.1	2.3	2.5	2.7	2.9	3.1	3.3	3.5	3.7	3.9	4.1	4.3
4.0 15	4.4	4.9	5.3	5.8	6.2	6.7	7.1	7.6	8.0	8.5	8.9	9.4	9.8
5.0 12	5.7	6.3	6.9	7.5	8.1	8.7	9.3	9.8	10.4	11.0	11.6	12.2	12.8
Dancing													
Moderately (waltz)	3.1	3.5	3.8	4.1	4.5	4.8	5.1	5.4	5.7	6/0	6.4	6.7	7.0
Active (square, disco)	4.5	5.0	5.4	5.9	6.3	6.8	7.3	7.7	8.2	8.6	9.1	9.5	10.0
Aerobic (vigorously)	6.0	6.7	7.3	7.9	8.5	9.1	9.7	10.3	10.9	11.5	12.1	12.7	13.3
Fencing													
Moderately	3.3	3.6	4.0	4.3	4.6	5.0	5.3	5.7	6.0	6.3	6.7	7.0	7.3
Vigorously	6.6	7.3	8.0	8.7	9.4	10.0	10.7	11.4	12.1	12.7	13.4	14.1	14.8
Football													
Moderate	3.3	3.6	4.0	4.3	4.6	5.0	5.3	5.7	6.0	6.3	6.7	7.0	7.3
Touch, vigorous	5.5	6.1	6.6	7.2	7.8	8.3	8.9	9.4	10.0	101.6	11.1	11.7	12.2
Golf													
Twosome (carry clubs)	3.6	4.0	4.4	4.7	5.1	5.4	5.8	6.2	6.6	6.9	7.3	7.6	8.0
Foursome (carry clubs)	2.7	3.0	3.3	3.5	3.8	4.1	4.4	4.6	4.9	5.2	5.4	5.7	6.0
Power-cart	1.9	2.1	2.3	2.5	2.7	2.9	3.1	3.3	3.5	3.7	3.9	4.1	4.3
Handball													
Moderate	6.5	7.2	7.8	8.5	9.2	9.9	10.5	11.2	11.9	12.5	13.2	13.8	14.5
Competitive	7.7	8.4	9.1	10.0	10.8	11.5	12.3	13.1	13.9	14.7	15.4	16.2	17.0

APPENDIX B: APPROXIMATE CALORIC EXPENDITURE PER MINUTE FOR VARIOUS PHYSICAL ACTIVITIES*

| Body Weight in kilograms | 45 | 50 | 55 | 59 | 64 | 68 | 73 | 77 | 82 | 86 | 91 | 95 | 100 |
Body Weight in pounds	100	110	120	130	140	150	160	170	180	190	200	210	220
PHYSICAL ACTIVITIES													
Hiking, pack (3 mph)	4.5	5.0	5.4	5.9	6.3	6.8	7.3	7.7	8.2	8.6	9.1	9.5	10.0
Hockey, field	5.0	6.7	7.3	7.9	8.5	9.1	9.7	10.3	10.9	11.5	12.1	12.7	13.3
Hockey, ice	6.6	7.3	8.0	8.7	9.4	10.0	10.7	11.4	12.1	12.7	13.4	14.1	14.8
Horseback riding													
Walk	1.9	2.1	2.3	2.5	2.7	2.9	3.1	3.3	3.5	3.7	3.9	4.1	4.3
Sitting to trot	2.7	3.0	3.3	3.5	3.8	4.1	4.4	4.6	4.9	5.2	5.4	5.7	6.0
Posting to trot	4.2	4.6	5.1	5.5	5.9	6.4	6.8	7.2	7.6	8.1	8.5	8.9	9.4
Gallop	5.7	6.3	6.9	7.5	8.1	8.7	9.3	9.8	10.4	11.0	11.6	12.2	12.8
Jogging (see Running)													
Judo	8.5	9.3	10.2	11.0	11.9	12.8	13.6	14.5	15.4	16.2	17.1	17.9	18.8
Karate	8.5	9.3	10.2	11.0	11.9	12.8	13.6	14.5	15.4	16.2	17.1	17.9	18.8
Mountain climbing	6.5	7.2	7.8	8.5	9.2	9.8	10.5	11.2	11.8	12.5	13.1	13.8	14.5
Paddle ball	5.7	6.3	6.9	7.5	8.1	8.7	9.3	9.8	10.4	11.0	11.6	12.2	12.8
Racketball	6.5	7.1	7.8	8.4	9.1	9.8	10.4	11.1	11.7	12.4	13.0	13.7	14.4
Roller skating (9 mph)	4.2	4.6	5.1	5.5	5.9	6.4	6.8	7.2	7.6	8.1	8.5	8.9	9.4
Running (steady state)													
(mph) (min/mile)													
5.0 12:00	6.0	6.6	7.3	7.9	8.5	9.1	9.7	10.3	10.9	11.6	12.2	12.8	13.4
5.5 10:55	6.7	7.3	8.0	8.7	9.4	10.0	10.7	11.4	12.1	12.8	13.4	14.1	14.8
6.0 10:00	7.2	8.0	8.7	9.5	10.2	10.9	11.7	12.4	13.1	13.8	14.6	15.4	16.1
7.0 8:35	8.5	9.3	10.2	11.0	11.9	12.8	13.6	14.5	15.4	16.2	17.1	17.9	18.8
8.0 7:30	9.7	10.7	11.6	12.6	13.6	14.6	15.6	16.6	17.6	18.5	19.5	20.5	21.5

APPENDIX B: APPROXIMATE CALORIC EXPENDITURE PER MINUTE FOR VARIOUS PHYSICAL ACTIVITIES*

Body Weight in kilograms	45	50	55	59	64	68	73	77	82	86	91	95	100
Body Weight in pounds	100	110	120	130	140	150	160	170	180	190	200	210	220
PHYSICAL ACTIVITIES													
Running (steady state) (continued)													
(mph) (min/mile)													
9.0 6:40	10.8	11.9	12.9	14.0	15.1	16.2	17.3	18.4	19.5	20.6	21.7	22.8	23.9
10.0 6:00	12.1	13.3	14.5	15.7	17.0	18.2	19.4	20.7	21.9	23.1	24.2	25.4	26.7
11.0 5:28	13.3	14.6	16.0	17.3	18.7	20.0	21.4	22.7	24.1	25.4	26.8	28.1	29.5
12.0 5:00	14.5	16.0	17.4	18.9	20.4	21.9	23.3	24.8	26.3	27.8	29.2	30.7	32.2
Skating, ice (9 mph)	4.2	4.6	5.1	5.5	5.9	6.4	6.8	7.2	7.6	8.1	8.5	8.9	9.4
Skiing, cross-country													
(mph) (min/mile)													
2.5 24:00	5.0	5.5	6.0	6.5	7.0	7.5	8.0	8.5	9.0	9.5	10.0	10.6	11.1
4.0 15:00	6.5	7.2	7.8	8.5	9.2	9.9	10.5	11.2	11.9	12.5	13.2	13.8	14.5
5.0 12:00	7.7	8.4	9.2	10.0	10.8	11.5	12.3	13.1	13.9	14.7	15.4	16.2	17.0
Skiing, downhill	6.5	7.2	7.8	8.5	9.2	9.9	10.5	11.2	11.9	12.5	13.2	13.8	14.5
Soccer	5.9	6.6	7.2	7.8	8.4	9.0	9.6	10.2	10.8	11.4	12.0	12.6	13.2
Squash													
Normal	6.7	7.3	8.0	8.7	9.5	10.1	10.8	11.5	12.2	12.9	13.5	14.2	14.9
Competition	7.7	8.4	9.2	10.0	10.8	11.5	12.3	13.1	13.9	14.7	15.4	16.2	17.0
Swimming (yards/mi)													
Backstroke													
25	2.5	2.8	3.0	3.3	3.5	3.8	4.0	4.3	4.5	4.8	5.1	5.3	5.6
30	3.5	3.9	4.2	4.6	4.9	5.3	5.6	6.0	6.4	6.7	7.1	7.4	7.8
35	4.5	5.0	5.4	5.9	6.3	6.8	7.3	7.7	8.2	8.6	9.1	9.5	10.0
40	5.5	6.1	6.6	7.2	7.8	8.3	8.9	9.4	10.0	10.6	11.1	11.7	12.2

APPENDIX B: APPROXIMATE CALORIC EXPENDITURE PER MINUTE FOR VARIOUS PHYSICAL ACTIVITIES*

| Body Weight in kilograms | 45 | 50 | 55 | 59 | 64 | 68 | 73 | 77 | 82 | 86 | 91 | 95 | 100 |
Body Weight in pounds	100	110	120	130	140	150	160	170	180	190	200	210	220
PHYSICAL ACTIVITIES													
Swimming (yards/mi)													
Breaststroke													
20	3.1	3.5	3.8	4.1	4.5	4.8	5.1	5.4	5.7	6.0	6.4	6.7	7.0
30	4.7	5.2	5.7	6.2	6.7	7.1	7.6	8.1	8.6	9.1	9.5	10.0	10.5
40	6.3	7.0	7.6	8.3	8.9	9.6	10.2	10.9	11.5	12.2	12.8	13.5	14.1
Front crawl													
20	3.1	3.5	3.8	4.1	4.5	4.8	5.1	5.4	5.7	6.0	6.4	6.7	7.0
25	4.0	4.4	4.8	5.2	5.6	6.0	6.4	6.8	7.2	7.6	8.0	8.4	8.8
35	4.8	5.4	5.9	6.4	6.8	7.3	7.8	8.3	8.8	9.2	9.7	10.2	10.7
45	5.7	6.3	6.9	7.5	8.1	8.7	9.3	9.8	10.4	11.0	11.6	12.2	12.8
50	7.0	7.7	8.5	9.2	9.9	10.6	11.3	12.0	12.8	13.5	14.2	14.9	15.6
Table tennis	3.4	3.8	4.1	4.5	4.8	5.2	5.5	5.9	6.3	6.6	7.0	7.3	7.7
Tennis													
Singles (recreational)	5.0	5.5	6.0	6.5	7.0	7.5	8.0	8.5	9.0	9.5	10.0	10.6	11.1
Competition	6.4	7.1	7.7	8.4	9.1	9.8	10.4	11.1	11.8	12.4	13.1	13.7	14.4
Volleyball													
Moderate recreational	2.9	3.2	3.5	3.8	4.1	4.4	4.7	5.0	5.3	5.6	5.9	6.1	6.4
Vigorous, competition	6.5	7.1	7.8	8.4	9.1	9.8	10.4	11.1	11.7	12.4	13.0	13.7	14.4
Walking (mph) (min/mile)													
2.0 30:00	2.1	2.3	2.5	2.8	3.0	3.2	3.4	3.6	3.9	4.1	4.3	4.5	4.7
3.0 20:00	2.7	3.0	3.3	3.5	3.8	4.1	4.4	4.6	4.9	5.2	5.4	5.7	6.0

APPENDIX B: APPROXIMATE CALORIC EXPENDITURE PER MINUTE FOR VARIOUS PHYSICAL ACTIVITIES*

Body Weight in kilograms		45	50	55	59	64	68	73	77	82	86	91	95	100
Body Weight in pounds		100	110	120	130	140	150	160	170	180	190	200	210	220
PHYSICAL ACTIVITIES														
Walking														
(mph)	(min/mile)													
3.5	17:10	3.3	3.7	4.0	4.4	4.7	5.1	5.4	5.8	6.2	6.5	6.9	7.2	7.6
4.0	15:00	4.2	4.6	5.1	5.5	5.9	6.4	6.8	7.2	7.6	8.1	8.5	8.9	9.4
4.5	13:20	4.7	5.2	5.7	6.2	6.7	7.1	7.6	8.1	8.6	9.1	9.5	10.0	10.5
5.0	12:00	5.4	6.0	6.5	7.1	7.7	8.2	8.7	9.2	9.8	10.4	10.9	11.5	12.0
5.4	11:10	6.2	6.9	7.5	8.2	8.8	9.5	10.1	10.3	11.4	12.1	12.7	13.4	14.0
5.8	10:20	7.7	8.4	9.2	10.0	10.8	11.5	12.3	13.1	13.9	14.7	15.4	16.2	17.0
Water skiing		5.0	5.5	6.0	6.5	7.0	7.5	8.0	8.5	9.0	9.5	10.0	10.6	11.1
Weight training		5.2	5.7	6.2	6.8	7.3	7.8	8.3	8.9	9.4	9.9	10.5	11.0	11.5
Wrestling		8.5	9.3	10.2	11.0	11.9	12.8	13.6	14.5	15.4	16.2	17.1	17.9	18.8

Note: The energy cost, in calories, will vary for different physical activities in a given individual depending on several factors. For example, the caloric cost of bicycling will vary depending on the type of bicycle, going uphill or downhill, and wind resistance. Walking with hand weights or ankle weights will increase energy output. Thus, the values expressed here are approximations and may be increased or decreased depending upon factors that influence energy cost.

INDEX

201

ABOUT THE
AUTHORS

Ellen Coleman, RD, MA, MPH, is a registered dietitian and exercise physiologist in Riverside, CA. She is the nutrition consultant for The S.P.O.R.T. Clinic. Ellen is the nutrition columnist for *Sports Medicine Digest* and author of *Eating for Endurance*. She has completed the Ironman triathlon in Hawaii twice and numerous marathons and 200-mile bicycle races. Ellen received the 1994 Achievement Award from the Sports, Cardiovascular, and Wellness Practice Group (SCAN) of the American Dietetic Association. She has consulted with the Los Angeles Lakers basketball team and the Anaheim Angels baseball team.

Suzanne Nelson Steen, DSc, RD, is the Head of Husky Sports Nutrition Services at the University of Washington, Department of Intercollegiate Athletics, Seattle, Washington. Previously, she was Chair of the Graduate Nutrition Education Department at Immaculata College, Immaculata, Pennsylvania. She has also served as Clinical Director of the Weight and Eating Disorders Center at the University of Pennsylvania School of Medicine, Philadelphia, Pennsylvania. Dr. Steen was a consulting nutritionist to USA Wrestling and was a member of the nutrition advisory committee for US Swimming. Throughout her career, Dr. Steen has worked with many different athletic teams, and counseled both recreational and elite athletes. Dr. Steen's work with athletes has been published in numerous scientific articles, and book chapters. She is co-editor of *Nutrition for Sport and Exercise*, and co-author of *Play Hard Eat Right—A Parents' Guide to Sports Nutrition for Children*.